ABUNDANTLY WELL

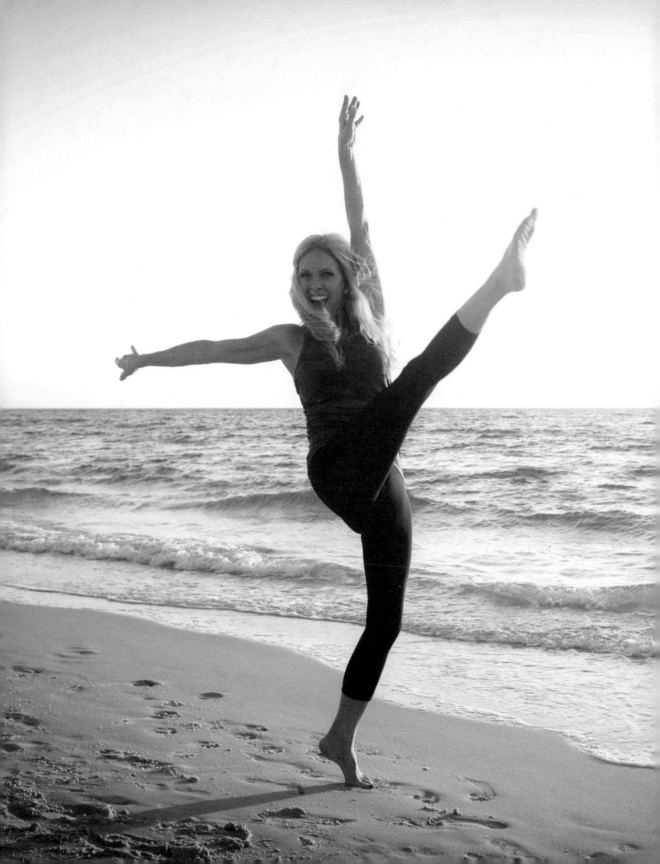

ABUNDANTLY WELL

BIBLE-BASED WISDOM FOR WEIGHT LOSS, INCREASED ENERGY, AND VIBRANT HEALTH

SHEMANE NUGENT

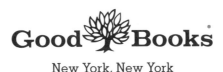

Good Books

New York, New York

Copyright © 2024 by Shemane Nugent

Photographs by Julie Renner, except photograph on page 160, which is by Bell Coleman

All rights reserved. No part of this book may be reproduced in any manner without the express written consent of the publisher, except in the case of brief excerpts in critical reviews or articles. All inquiries should be addressed to Good Books, 307 West 36th Street, 11th Floor, New York, NY 10018.

Good Books books may be purchased in bulk at special discounts for sales promotion, corporate gifts, fund-raising, or educational purposes. Special editions can also be created to specifications. For details, contact the Special Sales Department, Good Books, 307 West 36th Street, 11th Floor, New York, NY 10018 or info@skyhorsepublishing.com.

Good Books is an imprint of Skyhorse Publishing, Inc.®, a Delaware corporation.

Visit our website at www.goodbooks.com

10 9 8 7 6 5 4 3

Library of Congress Cataloging-in-Publication Data is available on file.

Cover design by Kai Texel
Cover photo by Julie Renner

Print ISBN: 978-1-68099-924-2
eBook ISBN: 978-1-68099-940-2

Unless otherwise marked, scripture quotations are from the ESV® Bible (The Holy Bible, English Standard Version®), © 2001 by Crossway, a publishing ministry of Good News Publishers. Used by permission. All rights reserved. The ESV text may not be quoted in any publication made available to the public by a Creative Commons license. The ESV may not be translated in whole or in part into any other language.

Scripture quotations marked (NIV) are taken from the Holy Bible, New International Version®, NIV®. Copyright © 1973, 1978, 1984, 2011 by Biblica, Inc.™ Used by permission of Zondervan. All rights reserved worldwide. www.zondervan.com. The "NIV" and "New International Version" are trademarks registered in the United States Patent and Trademark Office by Biblica, Inc.™

Printed in the United States of America

CONTENTS

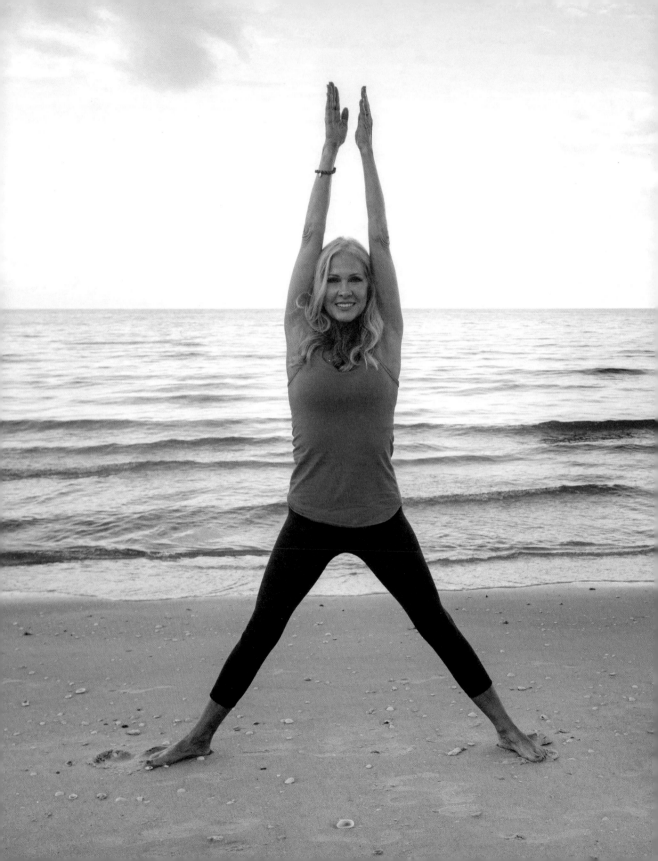

INTRODUCTION

"He gives power to the faint, and to him who has no might he increases strength." Isaiah 40:29

One spoonful of the velvety smooth, mint chocolate chip ice cream saved me from dying of heat stroke, or at least that's how I justified the cool, sweet treat. It was a scorching hot summer afternoon, and I had just come inside from cutting the grass with an old-fashioned push-mower. There was only one thing that could cool my body temperature quickly—ice cream.

Cutting the grass is hard work. I continued to shovel the satisfying deliciousness into my mouth, spoonful after spoonful. *I could have died from heat stroke. I was sweating profusely and I burned a few hundred calories, so it all evens out.*

A few moments later, the fear of heat stroke was long gone as I looked at the bottom of the empty ice cream carton. Guilt instantly replaced the satisfaction I had felt as I realized I had eaten the entire container.

I love to eat. I don't have a sweet tooth. *Every tooth* in my mouth savors ice cream, chocolate chip cookies, candy bars, cupcakes, apple pie, popcorn, pasta, pizza, Fritos, fried chicken, French fries . . . the list goes on. I have struggled with my weight all my life.

In college, I was thirty pounds heavier than I am now. The freshman fifteen was just the beginning. My diet included chocolate chip cookie dough for breakfast, cupcakes for lunch, and pizza for dinner. Then I'd starve myself for three days, existing on only Coke or Mountain Dew because I needed the caffeine for studying, and Rain-Blo bubble gum to curb my hunger pangs. Before there were sweatsuits made of plastic that really made you sweat, I wrapped my body in plastic wrap, put on a heavy cotton sweatsuit, and ran several miles. I inhaled a smorgasbord buffet, then tried to fast away my disgust and guilt.

I tried every diet I learned about from the cookie diet (of course), to the grapefruit diet (not a fan), to the blood-type diet, and everything in between. One of my prayers was, "God, please let me wake up tomorrow twenty pounds skinnier." As you can imagine, that prayer wasn't answered overnight.

For a decade I rode a roller-coaster ride of weight loss and gain. In my early twenties, after binging on a whole pizza followed by a few chocolate chip cookies, God showed me I needed to make significant changes to the way I was eating and what I ate. I was dishonoring God with my behavior and destroying his temple/my body according to 1 Corinthians 6:19. God showed me how to lose weight without starving, completely changing my lifestyle, or giving up Fritos and chocolate. How did I do it?

In *Abundantly Well*, I share the simple and incredibly effective techniques I applied to lose thirty pounds. Once I implemented those changes, I was able to release the pesky pounds that weighed me down and keep them off for thirty-five years—without missing out on birthday cake.

Exercise is a significant part of this health journey. If you've never worked out or despise going to the gym, don't worry. I'll show you how to get 'er done in less time and actually enjoy sit-ups.

As a fitness instructor for more than forty years, I've traveled the world sharing my passion for healthy living with hundreds of thousands of people. Everyone wants the same thing: to lose weight, tone muscles, and to have fun doing it. I don't want to do anything if it's not easy, effective, or fun, so I keep these pages short, sweet, funny, inspirational, and educational. In *Abundantly Well,* you'll see simple exercises sprinkled throughout this book that you can do for a few minutes a day, or you can string them together to make one complete, longer workout. It's your choice. Exercise is my number one secret to having less stress, minimizing inflammation, and aging gracefully.

What about wrinkles, arthritis, brown spots, joint pain, saggy skin, tooth decay and, um, bladder leakage? Those are certainly issues that don't often plague young adults, and we'll never have our twenty-year-old bodies again, but what if we *reimagine* the concept of aging to be the greatest, most exhilarating and sought-after experience of our lives?

The dark trials and tribulations we've endured provide us with insight and wisdom which are unavailable to younger people. What if wrinkles were appreciated, honored, and respected? What if we could really discover the fountain of youth and play tennis when we're eighty-five? Can we *redefine* misconceptions about being abundantly healthy at any age, and the possibility that the longer we live, the *greater* we live? If we *reframe* our mindset and shift our perspectives, we'll see ourselves as God sees us: Perfect in his Son.

WHY THIS BOOK? WHY NOW?

I promised myself and God that if I found answers to my struggles with my weight and health, I'd be bold and brave and share what I've learned with others. The tribulations that have caused me the most pain in my life—my mess—becomes my message. "Do not withhold good from those to whom it is due, when it is in your power to do it," says Proverbs 3:27.

When I got sick and nearly died from toxic mold between the walls of my MTV Cribs home, I became an investigative sleuth to cure myself and my family. Dozens of doctors failed to help, so I utilized the wisdom and knowledge I gained from my own research. Maybe you're at the point where you're frustrated, diets haven't worked, doctors haven't helped, and you want answers, too.

During the Covid-19 pandemic, regular doctor visits were discouraged and we were forced to rely on our own resources for minor maladies. That got me thinking . . . why don't we do that all the time? What if we found answers in nature, without taking man-made chemicals or pharmaceutical drugs? What if we could be abundantly healthier and happier by swapping one or two bad habits with natural options that could transform our health, relieve joint pain, and add quality years to our lives?

YOUR STYLE, YOUR WAY

For forty days, let's go on a journey to take back our health without completely giving up our favorite foods or spending two hours a day in the gym. If you don't know where to start and you haven't exercised in years, don't worry. Start with small steps like going for a ten minute walk, then gradually increase the length of time, expand your stride, and walk more vigorously. It's as simple as that!

You'll discover new strategies for weight loss that fit your lifestyle. You've tried everything? We'll discuss the possibility that spiritual warfare may be a reason you're not healthier. Together we'll lean into scripture that supports health and wellness. "For I will restore health to you, and your wounds I will heal, declares the Lord," (Jeremiah 30:17).

Abundantly Well is designed to be an interactive tool you use when you're waiting in the school pick-up line, between loads of laundry, or in the quiet and calm mornings you set aside just for you. Write and draw on the pages. Use them for journaling and Bible study. Highlight passages that tug at your heart and whisper to you.

If you've had setbacks in your life, know it's never too late to start fresh and begin a new day. Every day you open your eyes and take a breath is an opportunity to reawaken your senses and live another day filled with potentially exciting adventures.

NO TIME?

You may think that you don't have the time or discipline to wildly transform your health. Yes, it can get overwhelming. There are days when I can come up with a dozen excuses for why I shouldn't work out. After all, the laundry is piling up, crusted dishes in the sink beg for attention, and there are errands to run. Those excuses, however, were minimized when I made another significant shift in my life. Rather than telling myself that going to the gym was selfish, I replaced that stinking thinking with, *I'm getting healthy and strong for God.* Taking good care of our bodies is not selfish. It's critical. And if you're just too busy, I'll help you find a few extra minutes to fit exercise into the pockets of your time.

Wherever you are in your health journey is where you should start. More than once, I've heard people say, "I have to get into shape before I take your fitness class." Start here. Start now. It's always a good time to make a positive transformational shift in your life. God loves you. He created our bodies with the ability to heal and rejuvenate. Good health facilitates a life where you do the things you enjoy with the people you love.

No matter where you find yourself in your health and fitness journey right now, this book is designed to be your companion and coach to a better level of wellness. Whether you run marathons or can't manage your stairs, each day in this 40-Day devotional is designed to help you feel better, gain energy, and minimize stress so you can sleep more deeply.

You've picked up this book because you are ready to experience improvements in your health and quality of life. And you are not alone. According to the American Psychological Association, about one-third of Americans have made a health-related New Year's resolution, indicating a desire to improve health behaviors.

Let's discover what's really causing those late-night binges or lack of motivation to exercise and how you can change limiting beliefs about yourself. Caution: While simple and easy steps are provided to move you toward better health, your progress will be unique to you. Each of us is beautifully and wonderfully made. We have different families, education, environments, and stress. This is *your* path. What you put into these next forty days is up to you.

Being sick brought me closer to God, and I vowed that when I regained my health I'd share my wellness tips. Regardless of where you are on your health and fitness journey, I want to be your cheerleader. I've helped hundreds of thousands of people all over the world adopt healthier habits, and I know I can help you, too.

Let's get started!

"Do not be conformed to this world, but be transformed by the renewal of your mind, that by testing you may discern what is the will of God, what is good and acceptable and perfect." Romans 12:2

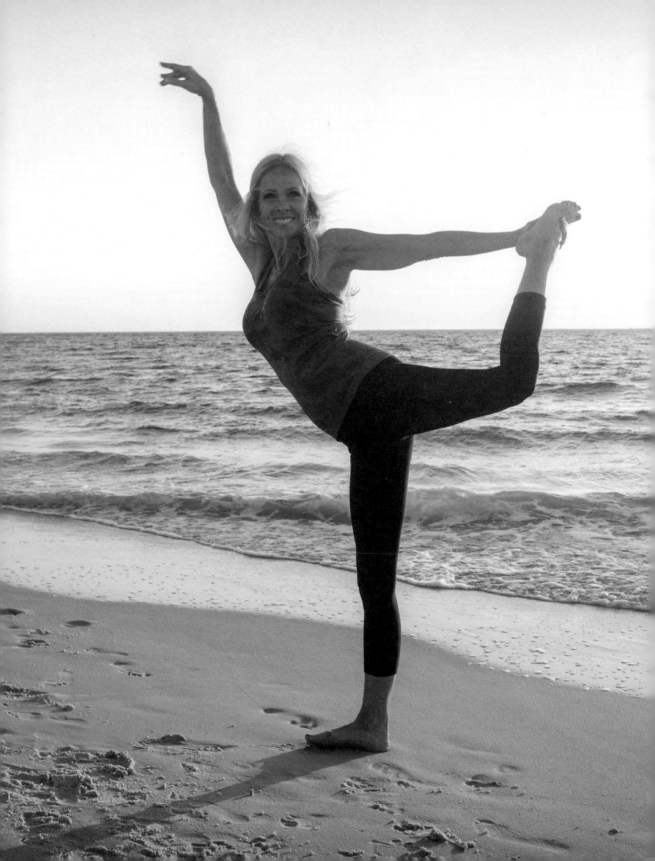

DAY 1
ASSESSMENT & DECLARATION

"I can do all things through him who strengthens me." Philippians 4:13

As a fitness instructor for more than forty years, I've seen the same types of people come into my exercise classes over and over.

The Superfit are the super healthy, marathon-running, perfectly chiseled, strong, energetic, fitness addicts who are committed and focused. They diligently track their cardio, strength training, and food intake. They drink pre- and post-workout formulated smoothies timed to boost their energy during their workouts, then aid in muscle repair and recovery after their time in the gym. They do not deviate from their schedules or cheat on their diets, and that's exactly why they are toned and sculpted.

To be honest, these workout pros make me want to step up my game in the gym. Like many, I can come up with a hundred excuses why I don't have time to exercise. The Superfit *make* time.

Moderately healthy individuals include exercise in their lives several times each week. They train hard in the gym and enjoy occasional indulgences. They eat salads and take vitamins, but don't deny themselves cupcakes and cookies and occasional beer and wine. I call them Weekend Warriors.

Sideliners are those who enjoy an occasional, leisurely bike ride or walk but are too busy, unwilling, or afraid to make the commitment to make their health a priority. Going to a gym can be daunting. Hundreds of complex-looking machines, treadmills, and medieval-looking exercise equipment can be intimidating. They've tried diets that don't work and became frustrated or bored with challenging workouts. Why bother? Plus, they're busy with work and family responsibilities. There's just no time. They're on the sidelines, waiting to get in the game, but rarely do.

Finally, there are those individuals who have given up on finding any redemption for their health. Perhaps they took vitamins, ate kale, and tried Pilates or CrossFit, but for too many reasons they decided weight loss and a healthier lifestyle were beyond reach.

You've heard the saying, "God does not give you more than you can handle." In my experience, there has been plenty that I couldn't come close to handling on my own. But when circumstances are more than I can manage, I'm reminded where my strength comes from. When I feel as though I want to give up, I lean into dependence on God.

To begin, evaluate where you are. Knowing where you are and where you want to go allows you to make a plan and celebrate your progress.

"WYA" is an acronym used in text messages to ask, "**W**here are **y**ou **a**t?" To make subtle or significant changes to your health, first determine the areas of your body/mind/spirit that need attention and prioritization with this health questionnaire.

- How much time do you exercise per week and for how long?
- On a scale of 1–10 (10 being the best), how healthy is your diet?
- Do you take supplements?

Holistically, let's assess your emotions, energy, and environment.

- Write about your wellness journey from childhood to now.
- Journal about what's holding you back from getting healthy.
- Determine the areas in your body/mind/spirit that need attention.
- Use the health questionnaire to prioritize what is most important.
- Sign the declaration that you will work toward getting healthier for 40 days.

1. TRANSFORMATION: EMBRACE HEALTH THROUGH SELF-ASSESSMENT AND DECLARATION

Through self-assessment, we identify hindrances like time and motivation that disappear before the unwavering belief in the transformative power of Christ as stated in 2 Corinthians 5:17: "Therefore, if anyone is in Christ, the new creation has come: The old has gone, the new is here." Take your first step toward a healthier life, break free from limitations, and embrace a new day of holistic well-being under the divine guidance of God.

ASSESSMENT

As you begin this forty-day quest for better health, let's get a baseline for where you are now. Respond quickly to the following questions without overthinking. The more honest you are, the easier it will be to reach your goals. For instance, if you say you don't struggle with late-night snacking (like I do), but at the end of these forty days you aren't seeing results, it might be because—a little tough love here—you're not owning what needs to change.

What happened in our past along with current lifestyle choices contribute to where we are right now. You've done the best you could with the trials and tribulations you've endured, so don't be hard on yourself. Now is the time to reimagine a brighter, healthier, and happier future. Rest assured, we aren't going to completely eliminate your favorite foods forever.

1. Physical Activity: How many times per week do you engage in exercise or physical activity?
   - Rarely or never
   - 1–2 times
   - 3–4 times
   - 5 or more times

What types of activity or exercise do you do most often? _____

On a scale of 1 to 10 (1 being light and 10 being intense), how would you rate the intensity of your exercise routine? _____

2. Health Issues: Which of these do you experience?
   A. Hypertension (high blood pressure)
   B. Diabetes
   C. Heart disease
   D. Osteoporosis
   E. Arthritis
   F. Cancer (specify type): _____
   G. Thyroid issues
   H. Respiratory conditions
   I. None of the above
   J. Other: _____

3. Emotional well-being: On average, are you:
   A. Happy
   B. Occasionally sad
   C. Sad
   D. Neutral
   E. Other: _____

Are there emotional wounds that may affect your current well-being?

Are there relationships in your life that are strained?

Do people often agitate you?

_____

_____

_____

4. Nutrition and diet: Describe your overall diet.
    A. Balanced and nutritious
    B. Mostly healthy with occasional indulgences
    C. Could be healthier
    D. Unhealthy

Is there a time of day or a particular environment when you lack discipline? Late night snacking, or snacking when driving?

_____

_____

_____

5. Sleep patterns
    - On average, how many hours of sleep do you get per night?
    - Do you keep electronics near your bed?
    - Do you watch TV or engage in social media at bedtime?
    - Do you often experience difficulty falling asleep or staying asleep?

_____

_____

_____

6. Lifestyle habits
    - How would you describe your physical activity level during the day? Sedentary, lightly active, moderately active, or very active?
    - Do you smoke? If yes, how much tobacco per day?
    - Do you consume alcohol? If yes, how often and in what quantities?

_____

_____

_____

7. Spirituality and faith
   - How often do you engage in prayer? Daily, during emergencies, or rarely?
   - Describe your relationship with God. Do you feel close, somewhat close, or distant?
   - Do you feel a sense of purpose and fulfillment in your life?
   - How often do you read the Bible? Daily, weekly, or almost never?

   _____

   _____

   _____

8. Goals: Would you like to:
   - ❏ Lose weight
   - ❏ Tone muscles
   - ❏ Improve flexibility
   - ❏ Have more energy
   - ❏ Sleep better
   - ❏ Be happier
   - ❏ Run a marathon or participate in another fitness competition
   - ❏ Have a better overall quality of life for as long as possible

9. Functional Medicine: Have you tried any of the following?
   - ❏ Infrared sauna
   - ❏ Vitamin IV
   - ❏ Oxygen therapy
   - ❏ Massage
   - ❏ Lymphatic drainage
   - ❏ HOCATT or hyperbaric chamber
   - ❏ EWOT (Exercise With Oxygen Therapy)
   - ❏ Fasting

10. Environment and Toxins
    - Do you use chemically scented soaps, detergents, or fabric softeners?
    - Has your home, vehicle, or office been flooded?
    - Has your house been tested for toxic mold?
    - Do you use chemically scented air fresheners?

    _____

    _____

Moving forward, this assessment provides a starting point and helps you see underlying issues that may prevent you from living abundantly well. At the end of your forty-day journey, take the assessment again and see your improvement.

Celebrate the small wins along the way. Have an attitude of gratitude and don't sweat the setbacks. We all have them. Together, we can do this!

DECLARATION

For the next forty days, and of my own free will, I make the choice to focus on improving my health. I pledge to spend approximately fifteen minutes reading one section per day. Some days I will have more time, others less. Exercise and healthy eating will be priorities, but my eyes will be fixed on God. I will listen to Him as much as I speak.

I'll lean into the recommended scripture and contemplate how it relates to me and my life. I may take notes in this book, or in my own journal. I might even memorize a few verses.

Most likely, I will falter once or twice and splurge on cupcakes or cookies, and that's okay. This program is about progress, not perfection.

I'll share some or all of my steps with family, friends, or on social media, with the intention of bringing others aboard this abundantly well ship that's about to set sail.

I am excited for the small wins—a lost pound or two, stronger muscles, and better sleep. Knowing that I can do all things through Christ who strengthens me will be the wind in my sail and peace in my heart.

_____

Signed, date

MOVE FORWARD

Take the assessment before moving on to the next day. At the end of your 40 days, take the assessment again and compare your before and after results.

PRAYER

Heavenly Father, thank you for this gift of life. My health is a precious treasure. Give me discipline in my food choices and the wisdom to know what my body needs to become healthier and stronger. May I embrace a more virtuous lifestyle that results in energy, peace, and vitality knowing that you are with me and will not leave me. As I begin this journey toward being abundantly well, I surrender my worries to you. I ask that any physical ailments and discomforts I'm experiencing right now leave my body. Provide me with radiating health and inner joy. In Jesus's name, amen.

DAY 2
SUPERNATURAL HEALTH

"Beloved, I pray that all may go well with you and that you may be in good health, as it goes well with your soul." 3 John 1:2

I f we believe the Bible to be true, we must acknowledge supernatural healing. There is a profound significance in treating our bodies as temples of the Holy Spirit, as stated in 1 Corinthians 6:19. Healthy physical activity maintains our body as a vessel of reverence and resilience. And then there are super moist, delicious cupcakes that make you feel like sunshine, or potato chips and the couch.

God gave us these amazing bodies that can jump and dance and swim, and sometimes we forget that our bones can break and we can't eat cupcakes like we did when we were kids. The older we get, the more we realize that we can choose to neglect our health or to take good care of this gift we've been given. Good health today impacts the quality of life we have tomorrow. And while there are things you or I cannot control—like the toxic mold illness that nearly killed me—we can grab some carrot sticks and nuts instead of the chips and start practicing good habits that enhance our health. Minor changes can have a huge impact.

According to dictionary.com, the definition of *supernatural* is "relating to, or being above or beyond what is natural; unexplainable by natural law or phenomena; abnormal." And ". . . attributed to God . . ." Health is a sacred gift from God, the embodiment of his divine strength, and a means to carry out his work. Feeling good and having energy can empower us to embrace and fulfill our God-given purpose. "For we are his workmanship, created in Christ Jesus for good works, which God prepared beforehand, that we should walk in them," Ephesians 2:10.

Having supernatural health combined with healthy spirituality is kind of like having a superpower. A 2015 study in the *Journal of Behavioral Medicine* found a positive relationship between religious belief and self-rated health.[*] An important part of supernatural healing is trusting our gut feeling, that inner wisdom, the power of your discernment, not logical thinking.

---

* Harold G Koenig, "Religion, Spirituality, and Health: The Research and Clinical Implications," ISRN psychiatry, December 16, 2012, https://www.ncbi.nlm.nih.gov/pmc/articles/PMC3671693/.

This is a gray area of spirituality that has recently gained popularity among doctors and psychologists, although philosophers such as Aristotle, Plato, Jung, and others have discussed it for centuries.

Our intuition and instincts are often spiritual connections and guidance from God. Have you ever felt a deep discomfort in a particular setting? Perhaps you're at a party or casual gathering and you have a sense that something is wrong, like watching a scary movie and suddenly there's dramatic music. Whitetail deer are typically brown in color. When danger is detected, the deer lifts its tail to reveal white markings and to signal other deer. Dogs are good at determining threats as well. Law enforcement, the military, boxers, and athletes use a heightened sense of awareness as discernment to direct their actions. Perhaps their blood pressure becomes elevated and their heart rate increases. We may not ever know why something felt unsafe, but when we listen to what our bodies are trying to tell us, we usually don't regret acting on that inner wisdom. Have you ever had an instinct to drive on a different road than normal, then realize you avoided a traffic jam? Those who ignore their intuition often say later they knew they should have chosen a different path but dismissed the feeling.

By delving into the concept of supernatural health and spiritual wisdom, we begin to trust those intuitive nudgings in our spirit, help others, and use our gifts and talents to serve God. We align our well-being with the aspirations of 3 John 1:2, where spiritual prosperity and vibrant health intertwine with our soul's divine purpose.

For anyone who has had a life-threatening illness or endured a traumatic situation, we have a subtle assurance that God has worked supernaturally in our lives. If you've experienced a situation where you defied the odds of survival, you'll likely have a grasp on what supernatural means. Maybe you were in an accident and the car was totaled but you walked away unscathed. Or perhaps a child with a terminal illness was healed and made a full recovery.

There are many scenarios where the worst imaginable outcome was replaced by something that could only be attributed to an unnatural phenomenon—to God—and we are forever changed. "Truly, truly, I say to you, whoever believes in me will also do the works that I do; and greater works than these will he do, because I am going to the Father. Whatever you ask in my name, this I will do, that the Father may be glorified in the Son. If you ask me anything in my name, I will do it," John 14:12–14.

Having supernatural health is to possess vitality to fight evil, heal the sick, cast out demons, and survive the coming storms with the peace of God. Jesus said, "For the Father loves the Son and shows him all he does. Yes, and he will show him even greater works than these, so that you will be amazed," John 5:20. We have things to do, people to heal, and loved ones to care for. We need divine intervention and the supernatural health and healing that only God can provide.

MOVE FORWARD

If you struggle with your health, God is your source for freedom to live an abundantly well, energized, and exciting life. Reimagine where you will be, physically, emotionally, and spiritually in forty days.

PRAYER

Father, thank you for a heart that beats, a body that moves, and for your gift of peace that surpasses all understanding. Thank you for my health. You are my Lord and Savior. I seek your face in the midst of turmoil. As Jesus said, greater works I can do. Fill me with supernatural health and peace. In Jesus's name, amen.

DAY 3
G.E.A.R.

Even to your old age and gray hairs
I am he, I am he who will sustain you.
I have made you and I will carry you;
I will sustain you and I will rescue you. (NIV)

For a few years after my toxic mold diagnosis, I focused on full recovery from the illness that nearly killed me. When Ted's tour took us to Las Vegas where he was booked to play several concerts, I challenged myself to attend a fitness class. A nearby health club offered exercise classes in Spinning and Step, which I had taught before I became ill. When I saw they also offered Zumba, a fitness class which involves cardio and Latin dance, a whisper of hopefulness entered my mind. *Could I do that?* Only a few months prior, I had been too weak to walk up a flight of stairs.

The instructor, Megan Gasper, glided across the wood floor dancing to salsa, merengue, cumbia, and hip hop music, engaging every participant with a huge smile. Minutes passed and my feet were still underneath me, my hips moving to the rhythm. I couldn't believe I had the energy to continue in such a high-energy workout. Sweating and grinning for the first time since becoming sick, I had come home to my familiar world of athletics and movement.

When you begin an exercise program, it is recommended that you consult with your doctor first. Next, make movement a habit, similar to common routines like brushing your teeth. Creating a routine happens over time. Get out of bed, brush your teeth, go to the bathroom, wash your hands and face, have coffee, work, make dinner, do household chores, tuck kids into bed. Rinse. Wash. Repeat. It's easier to have the same behaviors—even when they're potentially damaging—than to change. While one-third of Americans make New Year's resolutions, only 9 percent actually keep them.[*]

Change is hard. Disciplining ourselves to get out of our comfort zones can be physically and emotionally exhausting. The little voice in our head argues, *You've worked hard all your life. Why bother getting in shape now? There's a new season of your favorite show. Order pizza, have a glass of wine, and relax. You deserve it.*

---

[*]   "Society," YouGov, accessed October 21, 2023, https://today.yougov.com/topics/society/articles-reports.

You have made a resolution to improve your health. G.E.A.R. is an acronym to help you succeed in replacing a sedentary lifestyle with movement that keeps you abundantly well.

Get Ready:
- Schedule at least three days each week to include a thirty- to sixty-minute workout. If you exercise at home, choose an area that has at least eight square feet to move and groove. If you go to a gym, check the group fitness schedule for a class that looks interesting, fun, and challenging. Get together with a friend to walk and pray, or dance in a Zumba class. Friends can enhance the time, plus you'll have an accountability team.
- Set out your clothes, shoes, and water bottle the night before and be less rushed in the morning. Going for a run? Get your playlist ready.

Equip Yourself:
A great workout doesn't have to cost a lot of money. Use your own bodyweight for strength training. Good running shoes can cost less than thirty dollars at an outlet store. Whether exercising at home or at a gym, you will want to wear comfortable clothing that you can easily move in. Prioritize these items:

- Supportive running shoes
- Yoga mat for stretching, warm-up, and cool-down
- Water bottle

If you're working out at home, you may want to get a few supplies to maximize your training.

Basic Equipment
- Heavy, medium, and lightweight dumbbells
- Resistance bands

Intermediate Equipment
- Gliding discs
- Kettle bell
- Pilates ball (small)
- Stability ball (large)
- Step

Advanced Equipment
- Exercise bike
- Treadmill

- Rowing machine
- TRX
- Ballet bar

Attitude:

Positive Mindset: Set a positive intention for your workout. Visualize success and focus on how great you'll feel afterward.

Mindfulness: Practice mindfulness techniques such as deep breathing to clear your mind and reduce stress.

Set a Goal: Decide on the purpose of your workout, whether cardio, strength, flexibility, or a combination. Some days you will have more energy than others. Be kind to yourself when you don't feel energized. Showing up is the biggest step.

Routine: Which exercises you do are important, too. Include a warm-up and cool-down every time you exercise.

Warm-Up: Begin with moderate movement such as shoulder rolls followed by large arm circles. A dynamic warm-up includes gentle pulses or bounces that send your body the signal that you're getting ready for more. It brings blood flow throughout your body and lubricates your joints. Example: With a slight bend to your knees, lean your upper body forward and place your hands on your thighs. In this position, stick out your bum and lengthen your torso. Then, slowly arch your back and open the chest to form a C curve with your back. Repeat slowly.

Exercise Plan: Follow a structured workout routine that includes a mix of cardio, strength, and flexibility exercises. (See Workouts, page 139.)

Cool Down: End with a cool-down routine that includes gentle stretching to return your heart rate to normal and prevent muscle soreness.

MOVE FORWARD

Selecting new workout equipment can be fun! Treat yourself to colorful hand weights, gliding discs, or resistance bands. Getting new gear can be the incentive for you to get started on this abundantly well journey.

PRAYER

Thank you, Lord, for this body that moves. For the miraculous ways my muscles and joints work together. Guide my steps to make exercise a daily part of my life. I want to honor you with the body you gave me. Please provide strength, discipline, and an abundance of energy and stamina to get through this workout today. In Jesus's name, amen.

DAY 4
GET MOVING

"For while bodily training is of some value, godliness is of value in every way, as it holds promise for the present life and also for the life to come." 1 Timothy 4:8

"What is the best exercise to do?"

This is a common question posed to health and wellness coaches. The answer is, the best exercise is the one you will do. Developing a lifestyle that includes frequent moving of your body is far more important than choosing one "best" exercise that doesn't get done.

In the summer of 1991, *Three's Company* star Suzanne Somers introduced the Thigh Master, which guaranteed to tone your quadriceps and inner thighs. Along with millions of others, I bought one and used it every day *for a week*. Then, along with millions of others, I put the thigh master in the closet. Tae Bo became a nationwide phenomenon. Combining boxing, aerobics, and high intensity dance music, Billy Blanks was both motivational coach and a fit TV star. When I took Billy's Tae Bo class in Los Angeles, the facility was jam-packed like it was a rock concert. And when Billy walked onto the stage, all the girls in the room grinned and clapped. The energy was intense and exciting. I may have even kicked a little higher myself.

Spinning first started appearing on gym schedules in the nineties. One of the hardest workouts I ever did was when Spinning creator Johnny G taught the entire class standing next to me. He could see when I was challenging myself by increasing the tension on the stationary Schwinn bike, or wimping out by turning down the resistance.

After teaching thousands of people in thousands of classes from step to Spinning to kickboxing, my favorite workout is the program I helped develop, Zumba® in the Circuit. You can get a full body workout in sixty minutes and have fun dancing in the process, but that's not all I do.

To achieve a healthy, strong, and injury-proof body, I vary my workouts. If I'm short on time, I do High Intensity Interval Training (HIIT) or a Tabata workout. Both can be very intense, but they can also be modified for any level. Tabata, created by Japanese professor Dr. Izumi Tabata, is a form of HIIT, with a few differences. Tabata has a standard protocol where one particular exercise is performed at an all-out effort for twenty seconds, followed by a brief ten-second rest. Then repeat that cycle eight times. Tabata usually includes calisthenic-type exercises like jumping jacks and push-ups, but you can get creative and combine two exercises. For example: high jumps in place, then push-ups (burpees) for one Tabata set. Then bicep curls and overhead presses for another. HIIT rounds can vary in time, from thirty seconds to three minutes for the work period, and ten seconds to one minute to rest.

Seasons and preferences change. The sport that you liked to engage with previously may no longer hold your interest. Lifestyle changes affect the amount of time available to exercise, accessibility to resources, and even ability. Consistently vital is that we move our body daily and use our joints.

The best protection against aging is a body that stays in motion, keeping ligaments supple. Common exercises include walking, hiking, biking, skating, dancing, horseback riding, aerobics, golf, weightlifting, swimming, rowing, and yoga. Consider ping-pong, gardening, housework, or jump rope and hopscotch with the kids or grandkids. Get on a team to play basketball, baseball, volleyball, soccer, flag football, pickleball, or tennis.

The best preventative measure to guard against illness is to get in shape and stay healthy. According to the American Heart Association, less than 20 percent of women meet the Federal Physical Activity Guidelines.[*] Similarly, The Centers for Disease Control and Prevention states that just over 23 percent of US adults meet the Physical Activity Guidelines for both aerobic and muscle-strengthening activity.[†]

Now is the time to move your muscles and bones toward better health. Listen to your body as you begin and continue a fitness program. The key to lifelong health, exercise lowers blood pressure and cholesterol, improves sleep, reduces stress, and prevents the inflammation which can cause disease. Additionally, movement is proven to:

- Enhance antioxidant responses
- Promote the activation of cellular activity
- Improve metabolic function
- Reduce arterial stiffness
- Reduce inflammatory and oxidative damage
- Increase antioxidant enzymes and nitric oxide availability
- Improve functional performance

The rituals and patterns we evolve into over the years, like coming home from work, sitting on the sofa, and watching television, have created a certain neurological pathway that's familiar and difficult to revise. It's stuck in that cold, hard taffy phase. If you haven't exercised

---

[*]   "Physical Activity," www.heart.org, June 2, 2023, https://www.heart.org/en/get-involved/advocate /federal-priorities/physical-activity.

[†]   "Products—Data Briefs—Number 443—August 2022," Centers for Disease Control and Prevention, August 30, 2022, https://www.cdc.gov/nchs/products/databriefs/db443.htm#:~:text=In%202020%2C %2024.2%25%20of%20adults,for%20both%20men%20and%20women.

in months or years, embarking on a new fitness program will be daunting. The monkey in your mind argues, "You'd look silly walking into a gym," or "You don't know what you're doing." That monkey in your mind usually wins, doesn't she?

Even if you have not been physically active, you can start at any age. If you have a preexisting condition that prevents you from enjoying certain activities, begin where you are. Instead of looking at what you cannot do, focus on what you can.

WHERE TO BEGIN

You've faced challenges, haven't you? Your heart has been broken, smashed, stomped on, and chopped up. Pieces scattered everywhere. Maybe you just want to throw in the towel and quit. Don't. You. Dare. God isn't finished with you yet. In fact, He's just getting started!

Think about who you were ten or twenty years ago. Have you grown emotionally? Spiritually? Of course you have. You've weathered some significant storms you may not have ever thought you could endure. Losing ten or twenty pounds is nothing compared to losing a loved one. Some days will be easier and kinder than others. God is carefully shaping you into a warrior who is physically strong and emotionally prepared to fight spiritual warfare. You were born for such a time as this!

Remember the story of Esther in the Bible? She lost both of her parents and was sent to live with her uncle Mordecai. Selected as a potential wife to King Xerxes, she went through a year of beauty treatments and self-care. A year! My friend, your transformation can start right now. Imagine where you can be in a year!

Where do you start? With the next good and right thing. Begin with small and simple changes—movement you can do practically anywhere, even on an airplane.

During a five-hour cross-country trip, I heard flight attendants counting to twenty; then there would be silence and they would walk around the cabin assisting passengers. I'd hear them counting again to twenty, then it would stop.

They were behind the galley walls, so I couldn't see what they were doing. Strategically, I timed my bathroom break while they were counting. They were doing squats! Twenty squats, five times throughout the flight, equaled one hundred squats. Kudos to those flight attendants for creating a healthy work environment.

Squats done properly can help improve your health by jump-starting your metabolism. Such movements engage the body's largest muscle group and require oxygen intake, which speeds up the metabolic waste expulsion. Squats help with balance and are great exercises to tighten and tone the lower body.

Here are a few tips to do squats properly:

1. Stand with your feet shoulder-width apart.
2. Keep your back in a neutral position, and keep your knees centered over your feet.

3. Slowly bend your knees. Look in a side mirror to make sure your knees stay centered over your feet while you press your hips toward the back of the room.
4. Lower your hips as if you were about to sit into a chair.

Try doing four minutes of squats today. Repeat at least once a week. Check your progress in sixty days. How many squats can you do in four minutes?

MOVE FORWARD

Commit to exercising at least three times a week for a minimum of twenty minutes. Mix up your workouts. Vary the frequency, duration, and intensity.

PRAYER

Father God, thank you for loving me and offering me hope. Forgive me for all the times I've neglected to move my body when I know I should. I love you and know that your plan is better than my own. I have faith that you will restore my body with supernatural health, energy, and stamina. In Jesus's mighty name, amen.

DAY 5
HOME OR GYM

"Or do you not know that your body is a temple of the Holy Spirit within you, whom you have from God? You are not your own?" 1 Corinthians 6:19

.

The Superfit discussed in Day One are not just genetically blessed with abs of steel or thighs like Carrie Underwood's. They work very hard to stay in shape. Sure, there are Spanx to hold in your stomach and smooth bulges and many women wear them. Decades ago, women wore girdles, and before that corsets. Now, there are filters that sculpt the waist or remove wrinkles. But those are usually minor tweaks. A chiseled midsection or thighs like Carrie's takes diligence, determination, and discipline. Guess what? You can be in the Superfit club, too!

The main difference between Carrie's thighs and mine is time. She adheres to an unwavering strategy that includes many more minutes on leg extensions, squats, and lunges than I do. Plus, genetics and youth play a critical role. That said, we can all have better quadriceps, hamstrings, biceps, or triceps if we have one thing: motivation. Where do you get yours?

GYM WORKOUTS

It can be daunting to walk into a gym. Some of the machines look like medieval torture chambers and without the proper technique you could hurt yourself or someone else. Never feel embarrassed to ask for help. That's one reason you pay for a membership. If you're a people person, a gym membership could ignite a fitness fire within you. You'll meet new friends who are motivated to get healthy, and the best way to spark your drive to drop a few pounds is to surround yourself with others who have the same goals.

The staff at a gym or studio should be more than willing to offer advice about classes, equipment, and creating a successful plan that is right for you. That's why they're there. Don't hesitate to ask for suggestions. Is there a particular class or exercise they recommend based upon your previous workout history and any limitations or injuries you have?

Above all, listen for God's guidance when walking into a gym or studio. Do you feel upbeat, safe, and comfortable? Do you have friends who work out there?

January is the biggest month in the health club industry. People are inspired, at least for a couple of weeks, to lose the weight they gained the previous year, topped off by indulging in holiday festivities Thanksgiving through New Year's. Research indicates that less than 10 percent of people keep their New Year's resolutions.[*] Too soon, we lapse back into old habits.

When you consider health clubs in your area, take advantage of the free limited pass offered by gyms and specialty studios. For one day or one week, you can experience the facility and its amenities.

Here are things to consider when looking for the perfect place to invest your time, energy, and money:

- Is the gym clean?
- Is the staff friendly?
- Will they show you how to use equipment?
- Do they have childcare (if you need it)?
- Do they have a variety of group fitness classes?
- Are the instructors and trainers certified?
- What are their hours?
- What is their cancellation policy?
- Do they offer one private training session free?
- How many guest passes can you have?
- Will they give you a cash bonus for recommending a friend?
- Can you imagine yourself spending an hour or more each week at that facility?
- What are their amenities, such as sauna, pool, tanning, or massage?
- Is the location convenient?

Here's an inside tip: Sometimes there is wiggle room in the membership fee. It doesn't hurt to ask for the better rate.

HOME WORKOUTS

If you're on a tight budget or pressed for time, fear not. There are many options and benefits to working out at home. You don't have to worry about putting on makeup, if your workout clothes match, or about getting dressed and rushing out the door to be on time for a fitness class. However, at home, we can get distracted by kids, pets, and spouses. Are you able to focus on fitness for an hour when there are dishes in the sink, laundry to be done, and phone calls to make?

---

[*] Richard Batts, "Why Most New Year's Resolutions Fail: Lead Read Today," Lead Read Today | Fisher College of Business, February 2, 2023, https://fisher.osu.edu/blogs/leadreadtoday/why-most-new-years-resolutions-fail#:~:text=.

Online platforms offer a variety of physical conditioning sessions geared to different fitness modalities, length of workout, and type of music. Some charge monthly memberships while a variety of quality workouts are free. From Barre to Zumba, there's something for everyone. One drawback is that if you don't have prior knowledge of proper alignment when performing movements, you might not get the maximum benefit from the exercises or may even get injured. But the convenience of at-home workouts is a game-changer if you have fundamental exercise knowledge and can stay motivated to work out alone.

MY TAKE

Teaching group fitness classes makes me feel like sunshine. When I'm in front of eager exercise enthusiasts, I get a better workout because I can't just go through the motions. I have to reach higher and squat lower. It's also very therapeutic. My first job as an instructor is to make sure everyone is safe. *Is Susie bending her knees enough?* Then, I think about the choreography and my next move. *What's next, the step-touch? Is the music too loud?* My mind is filled with an immediate to-do list and there's no time for dwelling on a bad hair day. It lights up my spirit to see so many people dancing, sweating, and smiling.

If I'm not teaching, however, I usually exercise at home. Since I've been in the fitness industry for more than forty years and have either taught or tried nearly every type of workout, I know what I like and which exercises are most effective for me. I understand body alignment and when I'm pushing myself too hard, or not hard enough. I can choose a twenty-minute HIIT workout with music that inspires me, and one that will kick my butt.

My best advice is to create a hybrid training program that involves taking a few classes at a gym, working out regularly at home, and an occasional walking get-together with your spouse or with friends. If you can afford it, hire a personal trainer to get you started and create a program you can stick to. Oftentimes, trainers will agree to coach two or three people at a time to cut the cost.

Make fitness a priority in your life and you'll see amazing changes in your health, energy, and mindset.

MOVE FORWARD

Find a friend who you can exercise with once a week, or even once a month. It's fun to talk with a friend, and being with another person will help keep you accountable. You're less likely to skip the workout when you make a plan that involves accountability to someone else. It comes down to this: How bad do you want it? If time and money aren't deterrents, I'd highly recommend getting a membership at a local gym and weekly sessions with a qualified trainer.

PRAYER

God, I come to you humbly and grateful for this body. Forgive me for the ways in which I've neglected my health. I'm ready, God, to get in shape and exercise these weary bones. Show me the best ways I can stay motivated to get stronger and make fitness a part of my daily life. Put like-minded, faith-filled people in my life so we can encourage one another and be better stewards of our bodies. Help me to have discipline, and to find time to work out even when I'm not eager to. In Jesus's name, amen.

DAY 6
HEAL YOUR PAST TRAUMA

"He heals the brokenhearted and binds up their wounds." Psalm 147:3

The toxicologist reached into his white lab coat and pulled out his prescription pad. Carefully and slowly, he penned letters.

Great. More drugs.

He handed me the script. But instead of another medication, he wrote words that caught me entirely off guard.

Get out of the house.

I looked at him.

"It's simple." He pointed to the script. "Leave your home. Take no belongings. Don't look back."

Earlier, I located a toxicologist who had been doing extensive blood tests on the nine-eleven volunteers diagnosed with illnesses including asthma, rhinosinusitis, gastroesophageal reflux, chronic obstructive pulmonary disease, and cancer. The tests weren't cheap, but I had to find out what was killing me. I had to get them done.

When my results were ready, I made the trip back to Detroit to meet with the specialist. My body felt terribly weak as I tried to get comfortable on the exam table in the toxicology doctor's sparse office. Already feeling chilled, my blood ran cold to see the test results. My diagnosis included pre-emphysema, which explained the chest tightness, shortness of breath, and sensation that an elephant had chosen my chest as a place to sit. The report confirmed I had four different types of mold in my bloodstream including the deadliest, Stachybotrys.

How could four types of mold get into my bloodstream? The news hit like a Mike Tyson sucker punch. *What do I do now?*

Unquestionably, there is a physiological reaction that takes place in our bodies when we are sad, depressed, or feeling anxious. The stress of losing a loved one can lead to death. Broken heart syndrome, also called stress-induced cardiomyopathy, can weaken the immune system and make the body vulnerable to serious diseases.

When I discovered my husband's affair, I lost weight, couldn't eat, couldn't sleep, and couldn't focus on daily chores for months. Okay, years. My mind seemed to betray me, as I could only think about the red flags I missed. It felt like I was carrying a cement block around with me everywhere. I was exhausted.

Now, decades later, I realize that emotionally painful time occurred immediately prior to my life-threatening illness. Is it possible that the trauma weakened my immune system and opened the door to more destruction physically and mentally?

NOT ALONE

According to the National Survey of Children's Health, nearly 35 million US children have experienced one or more types of trauma.* We've all suffered from devastating disappointments and rejections. Things don't always happen as planned. Loved ones pass unexpectedly. There are victims of heinous crimes and unthinkable actions that forever darken our days and cause us to question our faith. Evil exists. The devil comes to steal your joy, take away (kill) your health, and destroy your faith. Past wounds may haunt us in ways that we can easily feel in our bodies years later. Resources such as *The Body Keeps the Score, The Deepest Well*, and *Boundaries for Your Soul* remind us that trauma impacts our mental and physical health. It's not unusual for scents and smells, sights and sounds, and aches in our bodies to trigger painful memories, and, conversely, for emotionally painful experiences to result in physical pain, even many years later.

A social media post by someone I've never met conjures up instant angst. She raves about her faithful husband and rock solid marriage and I instantly think, *I'll never have that*. So, I do my best to distract myself and move through the muddy mess—laundry, dishes, errands—until I catch a glimpse of sunlight peeking through the clouds. A sliver of hope and the hint of peace of mind.

"And after you have suffered a little while, the God of all grace, who has called you to his eternal glory in Christ, will himself restore, confirm, strengthen, and establish you," 1 Peter 5:10. When hope is lost, confidence wanes as well. With patience, prayer, and practice, we learn to reframe the event and interpret greater meaning. Deconstructing childhood dreams that haven't come to fruition, a midlife crisis, or a general feeling of discontentment can eventually spark creativity and inspiration.

Looking back, I've learned so much from losing my health and from trials in my marriage. I'm not the same person I used to be. And for that, I'm grateful.

Everyone reacts differently to stress. Some people throw their energy into longer work hours or more exercise. Others might curl up on the couch with a bag of chips. Emotional eating is often linked to disappointments or trauma we've experienced in our lives. Had a tough day at work? Eating cookies always seems to help, doesn't it?

---

* Jane Ellen Stevens, "Nearly 35 Million U.S. Children Have Experienced One or More Types of Childhood Trauma," ACEs Too High, April 25, 2017, https://acestoohigh.com/2013/05/13/nearly-35 -million-u-s-children-have-experienced-one-or-more-types-of-childhood-trauma/.

The transformative journey of healing from past trauma begins with prayer. The thing that brings us to our knees also brings us closer to God. It is His comforting presence that heals our broken hearts and binds our wounds. Powerful lessons can be learned from past mistakes. We can learn how to extend forgiveness and receive it. Though not a simple or quick process, it is through embracing these challenges as catalysts that we experience the deepest spiritual growth.

BOUNDARIES

Whenever we're triggered by a person or a situation there are options. One solution is to remove yourself calmly and quietly from a problematic environment. Give yourself grace and space. It's okay that we don't get along with everyone. Once I studied the Enneagram personality types and got over the shock of realizing how different each one of us really are, the whole world seemed to open, like the sun breaking through the clouds after a storm. Analytical people will interpret situations with less emotion and much differently from creative types who get teary-eyed easily. We are all flawed and imperfect people trying to do the best we can.

If, during conflict, someone reacts completely differently than you'd expect, try to remember they're dealing with their own trauma and stress. Say a quick prayer asking for guidance instead of allowing the energy in the room to become thick and tense. It's not easy to do, especially when someone betrayed you, or when you have deep differences, but the more you do it, the better you'll get. It's like jump roping. After stepping on the rope enough times, you'll eventually catch a rhythm.

"You shall not take vengeance or bear a grudge against the sons of your own people, but you shall love your neighbor as yourself," Leviticus 19:18. Setting boundaries for the next time you're in the presence of someone who upsets you can help ease your anxiety. For example, if you know that someone who's hurt or betrayed you is going to be at an event or activity you're attending, you can choose to keep your distance and focus on the main aspect of the get-together. Don't let someone ruin a nice day. You can't control what others say or do, but you can control your reaction.

Sometimes we overthink things, too. Or maybe that's just me. The devil wants us discouraged, frustrated, and angry, and when people push our buttons, we get that way more quickly. The key is to prevent or at least delay a contentious situation. Protecting your mindset is part of aging gracefully. Bite your tongue, change the subject, or find something positive to focus on. You can choose to experience victory rather than play the victim.

"He will wipe away every tear from their eyes, and death shall be no more, neither shall there be mourning, nor crying, nor pain anymore, for the former things have passed away," Revelation 21:4. And "And he who was seated on the throne said, 'Behold, I am making all things new,'" Revelation 21:5.

Many of us despise change. Think about something positive in your life, regardless of how meaningless it might seem. A brief morning walk with your dog when the birds are singing can be a beautiful start to your day. When we find ourselves thinking negatively and complaining often, those thoughts become predominant in our minds. 2 Corinthians 10:5 tells us to "take captive every thought to make it obedient to Christ," because thoughts create pathways in our brain. We can choose to focus on what is life-giving.

Do you have a minute? *Just one. Maybe two.* Take a walk outside and think about how you can *reframe your thinking* during unresolved conflicts. Getting outdoors or trying something new reminds us that the world is larger than our current frustration. For example: *Suzy just snapped at me. It's her job to get the reports done on time. Suzy just found out her mother has cancer. She probably didn't lash out at me intentionally. She's frustrated and scared.*

Breathe deeply and exhale. Visualize the tension in your body minimizing. Distract yourself with something else for a few minutes and extract from the situation. We can change our mindset when we *reframe* the situation. *I have a little extra time today. I can finish those reports for Suzy.*

Reframe rejection, setbacks, and disappointments to help determine what you really want and don't want in life. Throughout our lives, we've had good experiences and bad. Times that have brought us to our knees.

Describe one of those tribulations.

Describe the hurt and pain you experienced.

Can you *reimagine* something positive resulting from that experience? Little things add up. Imagine a frustrating situation when you lost patience and reacted harshly. You can *reimagine, redefine,* and *reframe* those situations to thwart a future outburst.

Describe a conflict in your life and how the situation makes you feel. Did your attitude or behavior change in some way for good? How can you become more peaceful during conflicts with others? What boundaries can you set to protect your emotional well-being?

MOVE FORWARD

Pretend you are holding a baby. You cradle the baby's head in the crease of your elbow. You smell that wonderful baby scent and you want to protect that baby from harm. Imagine yourself in that situation right now. Describe what you see and feel.

Now, imagine that baby is *you.* Describe the thoughts and emotions tied to protecting others from harm versus protecting yourself.

PRAYER

Heavenly Father, I come to you with a humble heart. There are things in my past that trouble and haunt me. Fill me with the calmness that only you can provide. Guide my attitude and steps to walk in peace today no matter what difficulties come my way. I break the chains that bind me to unforgiveness. In Jesus's name, amen.

DAY 7
GOD FOOD VERSUS MAN FOOD

"Every moving thing that lives shall be food for you. And as I gave you the green plants, I give you everything." Genesis 9:3

There's a "beef" about harvesting your own food versus paying someone else to provide you with plastic-wrapped portions of meat at the grocery store. As a bowhunter, I know how much time is spent preparing for one deer hunt. Unlike the guaranteed kill in slaughterhouses, there's no promise that sitting in a tree stand with a bow and arrow will result in dinner on the table. Months and years of practice and hours of preparation go into just one hunt. I sit and wait and sit some more. To be able to draw a bow with the eyes and ears of birds and squirrels and other wildlife on you is almost impossible. Plus, with bowhunting, the deer has to be within approximately twenty yards standing sideways—*with its front leg forward*. Having proficiency with a gun or a bow takes lots of patience, stealth, and practice. Even if you hit the bull's-eye every time, don't get the grill warmed up just yet.

Hunting, especially bowhunting, is not easy or quick, but it can be rewarding. Think of this: if you could only get your dinner by growing your own vegetables or killing a cow, a deer, a lamb, or a pig—could you do it? Not everyone is cut out to be a hunter, but if you really want to appreciate your chicken fried steak, meatloaf, or spaghetti bolognese, get it yourself.

Some people say they could never kill an animal, but even if you're a vegan, you are responsible for killing millions of birds, geese, rabbits, possums, and deer. The roads you drive on, the shopping mall you frequent, your house—these were all once wildlife habitat. Your vegetable garden too! By making way for those areas to be habitat-free, you have to kill every squirrel, rabbit, chipmunk, pheasant, dove, turkey, and deer. We are all complicit.

Most importantly, I believe, we're missing out on a crucial part of the equation: responsible stewardship. "Then God said, 'Let us make man in our image, after our likeness. And let them have dominion over the fish of the sea and over the birds of the heavens and over the livestock and over all the earth and over every creeping thing that creeps on the earth.'

"So God created man in his own image, in the image of God he created him; male and female he created them. And God blessed them. And God said to them, 'Be fruitful and multiply and fill the earth and subdue it, and have dominion over the fish of the sea and over the birds of the heavens and over every living thing that moves on the earth.' And God said, 'Behold, I have given you every plant yielding seed that is on the face of all the earth, and every tree with seed in its fruit. You shall have them for food. And to every beast of the earth and to every bird of the heavens and to everything that creeps on the earth, everything that has the breath of life, I have given every green plant for food.' And it was so. And God saw everything that he had made, and behold, it was very good. And there was evening and there was morning, the sixth day," Genesis 1:26–31.

Every year hunters pay for licenses to hunt. That money goes into protecting wildlife habitat. These renewable, God-given resources continue to grow in numbers. Each year, nearly every doe has one to three fawns. Yet we continue to build homes, shopping malls, and highways. As a result, there are over a million car-deer accidents every twelve months in America.[*] Sadly, that precious protein goes to waste on the side of the road. In states including Colorado, Texas, Maryland, Wisconsin, and Pennsylvania, tax dollars go to government paid hunters who help control deer, bear, and mountain lions at airports, on hiking trails, and near homes. That could be you with your bow and arrow getting venison that's not inoculated with growth hormones and antibiotics.

MODIFIED FOOD

The nineteen-sixties cartoon *The Jetsons* focused on a family living in a futuristic, technologically advanced world. With a push of a button, Jane Jetson instantaneously prepared well-balanced meals for her family. Growing up, we gathered around our TV and ate convenient, prepackaged or frozen dinners on TV trays and thought we were living the good life. My favorite was Hamburger Helper. Just add water and cooked meat.

Today, with 3D printers and genetically modified (GMO) food, we're getting even closer to the Jetson space age robotics. Next thing you know, there will be flying cars. It's almost scary to think that scientists today can extract a cell sample from an animal, grow it in a laboratory, and print it through a 3D printer.

While there are advantages to bioengineering food, like solving world hunger, there are more reasons to reject this Jetson modernization. Processed foods contain unnecessary additives, preservatives, food dyes, sugars, sodium, and carcinogens. Prepackaged foods might taste good, (remember Twinkies?), but they lack nutrients and essential vitamins, minerals, and antioxidants. They might be killing us, too.

A diet lacking in nutrient-dense foods can weaken the body's immune system and inhibit the ability to fight chronic diseases like diabetes and cancer. The term "GMO" has only been in our vocabulary and on store shelves for a few years. What are the long-term side effects

---

[*]   Nathan Paulus, "Deer Auto Collisions by the Numbers," MoneyGeek.com, February 13, 2023, https://www.moneygeek.com/insurance/auto/deer-car-accidents/#:~:text=.

from eating so-called food that doesn't have the essential vitamins and minerals? Grabbing a sandwich in sixty seconds from a drive-through window might seem easier and more convenient, but if you really knew all of the cancer-causing, obesity-creating ingredients that are in processed foods, the convenience is not a worthy trade.

Because of this age of convenience dining, we are setting ourselves up for a lifetime of chronic diseases. Our bodies—these sacred temples—were not made to ingest man-made, chemical-filled substances. Unconsciously, when we consume ultra-processed foods, we might eat an additional five hundred calories per day.[*]

Sugar lurks in many foods labeled as sucrose, fructose, and other natural-sounding ingredients, while contributing to weight gain, diabetes, high blood pressure, obesity, and many health problems. Sugar is the new tobacco, more addictive than cocaine.

Here are five steps to help break the sugar addiction:

1. **Don't eat what you can't pronounce.** Many products on grocery store shelves contain chemically processed additives that shouldn't be called food. The closer the food source is to the hoof, ground, or the tree, the better nutritionally. The less we process our food, the healthier it is. This goes for artificial sweeteners too. Aspartame causes migraines and other diseases, not to mention a horrible aftertaste.

2. **Become a label reader.** If the product is in a box on a shelf for months or years, is it the best fuel for your body? Sugar often hides in our favorite foods that wouldn't be considered dessert, from spaghetti sauce to catsup, soup, yogurt, and pizza. Soda contains 30 to 50 grams of sugar in a single can.

3. **Use the 80/20 rule.** Eighty percent of what I eat is darn healthy, clean, and organic. Twenty percent is reserved for chips and salsa or my homemade chocolate chip cookies on occasion. Life for me is about balance and not denying a few, minimal indulgences.

4. **Eat more vegetables.** Sugar cravings can be minimized by eating healthy snacks like carrots or cucumbers with a smidgen of hummus. These foods provide energy for our bodies.

5. **"Sugar is the devil"** is my mantra whenever I feel the urge to overindulge. Feel free to use it. Here is one way to look at it: The thief comes to steal your health, kill your mindset, and destroy your life (John 10:10).

A growing percentage of people are interested in becoming self-sufficient and living off the land. Many are concerned with flavor enhancers and stabilizers designed to prolong shelf-life. Some don't trust the government. Whichever way, when you procure your own sustenance, fewer chemicals equals better health.

---

[*] Jordan Liles, "About That 'Lucky Charms Are Healthier Than Steak' Food Pyramid," Snopes, January 18, 2023, https://www.snopes.com/news/2023/01/16/lucky-charms-healthier-than-steak-food-pyramid.

Besides the health risks of consuming man-made food that grows more quickly and colorfully, there are moral and ethical considerations. Religious guidelines for eating particular foods may be in question. Is 3D-printed meat considered kosher?

Caring for and cultivating your own source of food can provide a sense of peace in a technologically noisy world. Watching golden squash blossoms open in the early morning sun immediately alleviates feelings of anxiety and stress. Gardening includes the added health benefits of physical movement and exercise. When I pull weeds in my garden or pick peppers and snip fresh herbs from my own garden, I have a sense of accomplishment. I planted the seed, watered the soil, and watched it grow. Getting outdoors regularly for even ten minutes has a stress-easing impact on the body.

Growing our own food or hunting for our dinner slows us down and helps us appreciate God's miraculous design. No 3D printer can give that satisfaction.

Quick tips toward better health include:

- Avoid processed food
- Eat and/or drink vegetables often
- Make your diet primarily protein, vegetables, fruit, and whole grains
- Avoid monosodium glutamate (MSG), food dyes, and boxed food with preservatives
- Start a garden, if you haven't already
- Buy organic food whenever possible

MOVE FORWARD

Prior to eating anything else, have a few raw carrots or celery. Drink a glass or two of water with lemon slices added. Make dips of fresh guacamole, hummus, and refried beans to help quell sugar cravings.

PRAYER

Father God, we come to you grateful for your sacred gift of sustenance. Protect our ranchers, hunters, and farmers—those responsible stewards and conservationists who produce natural and wholesome nourishment. Help me to appreciate the blessing and abundance of food that is readily available. In Jesus's name, amen.

DAY 8
LESS IS MORE

"If you have found honey, eat only enough for you,
lest you have your fill of it and vomit it." Proverbs 25:16

Growing up, my nickname was Shelly. Occasionally, kids called me, "Shelly with the big, fat belly." During my school years, I was involved in many sports and people described me as "healthy" or "big-boned." I prayed I would be as skinny as the models on magazine covers.

Though as a family we occasionally had fancy dinners with crystal and china after church, most nights the main course was Hamburger Helper, chicken pot pies, or frozen dinners. During junior high and high school, my packed lunch frequently consisted of a peanut butter and jelly sandwich, bag of chips, and two Hostess cupcakes.

It wasn't until I reached voting age and my high school sports days were long gone that I understood the effect food had on my body. I was no longer burning off the calories in competitive swimming, track, volleyball, basketball, or gymnastics. The cupcakes and Twinkies were finally catching up with me.

Exercise and healthy eating are responsible for overall health and wellness. Yes, genetics plays a role. I'll never be five foot eleven while weighing one hundred and ten pounds. For one thing, I like to eat. (I may or may not have had two homemade chocolate chip cookies while writing this day's text.) But I've figured out how to maintain my body weight and size for thirty years. Except that one time . . .

After having a hysterectomy to remove a significantly-sized tumor, my fifty-year-old body was finally slowing down. For months after the surgery, I could barely get through the day without extra caffeine. For the first time in my life, I had no energy *and I was gaining weight!* Although I knew all the tricks to fit into my Mother jeans (starving, Saran Wrap, and saunas), nothing worked as it had before. Tossing gas on the fire, I had been hired to be the co-star in a workout video for Zumba. In a few months, I would be traveling the world as an International Zumba fitness presenter—on stage in front of thousands of instructors.

So I tried something new: for one week, I ate smaller portions of meat, healthy oils, and only slightly cooked vegetables. No carbs. Daily I had a palm-sized portion of fish, chicken, or venison, healthy fats such as avocados, extra virgin olive oil, and nuts for snacking. No fruit, potatoes, bread, or rice. The result: My energy shot through the roof. I felt better than I had in years. As a side effect, my cravings for sweets diminished too.

Some doctors may disagree, and I'm not saying this is the right nutrition plan for everyone, but it worked for me for a short period of time. For the past few years, I've been on a modified version of this, sticking basically to a ketogenic diet while allowing occasional treats—*hence the chocolate chip cookies.* It's important that you consult your doctors about the proper nutrition plan for you.

We seldom eat enough vegetables, and yet the green stuff can be the most nutrient-rich food with which we can fuel our bodies. By simplifying my diet to center around protein, vegetables, and healthy fats, with minimal complex carbs, I have been able to maintain my weight, while still allowing a small piece of chocolate or chocolate chip cookie every day. Living a life focused on health and maintaining a healthy weight is far easier than crash dieting to drop 20 pounds before a wedding, class reunion, or summer bathing suit season.

Rather than counting calories, try looking at the bigger picture. Eat 80 percent naturally wholesome foods that fuel your body, while reserving that 20 percent of your intake for a burger (with the bun), chips and salsa, or your aunt's lasagna. It makes decisions around food easier, without stressing about being "perfect."

MORE OUTDOORS

Sometimes we obsess about what to eat or how much (or maybe that's just me). At breakfast, we start thinking about what we'll have for dinner. We say we're only going to have one potato chip and then can't stop thinking about the rest of the bag. Whenever I feel pulled to eat more than I know I should, or I become infatuated with food choices, I take a walk. Less time indoors and more time outdoors has healing and rejuvenating effects on your mind, body, and soul.

There is nothing more peaceful than being surrounded by nature and enveloped by its healing power. The sight of colorful birds and trees, the symphonic sound of crickets and birds, the gentle kiss of wind on your face, and the smell of freshly cut grass or a fragrant gardenia can be an instant stress reducer. And suddenly, I forget about food! It's also the perfect opportunity to spend time with God.

Have you ever gone for a walk to clear your head and suddenly come up with creative thoughts about how to solve a problem or design something new? Inspiration takes place in many forms and in many places. Being in nature can do more than just enhance our sense of vitality. It can be prayer time, too.

When I was hospitalized for migraines, a neurologist suggested I listen to recorded sounds of nature in a dark room. *Why not just go outside?* At that point, I realized breathing fresh air was more than just a temporary fix to relieve stress, but also innately rewarding. To fully envelop yourself in God's creation is energizing and enlightening. If you've never watched the sun dip into the horizon until it's completely disappeared, you simply must.

Earthing is a medical term that involves feeling the earth's energy beneath your feet. Rubber- or leather-soled shoes prevent the earth's vibration from touching our hands or feet.

Numerous studies indicate a positive response among individuals who routinely get in physical touch with the earth. My happiest times are when I'm walking on the beach barefoot. It feels peaceful and rejuvenating and I always come away refreshed.

Less screen time, recycled air, and modified foods and more silence, food from the ground, and connection with nature is a formula for better health. Sleep improves and our weight more easily settles to what is healthiest for our body. Want to get more out of your workout? Take it outside. Research shows that exercising outdoors can enhance your self-esteem and lead to a greater sense of well-being. Take a few minutes today to enjoy and celebrate the spirit of the wild.

MOVE FORWARD

If only for today, minimize your meals to palm-sized portions. Minimize foods and drinks with sugar. Get outdoors even for ten minutes.

PRAYER

Heavenly Father, I'm grateful for the opportunity to begin a new day, in a new way. Send your Holy Spirit as my helper and my guide to be satisfied with eating less. I break the spirit of gluttony in Jesus's mighty name, amen.

DAY 9
FASTING

"Is not this the kind of fasting I have chosen: to loose the chains of injustice and untie the cords of the yoke, to set the oppressed free and break every yoke?" Isaiah 58:6 (NIV)

The human body is filled with intricately organized cells, tissues, organs, and bones that work twenty-four hours a day, seven days a week to keep us alive. Our digestive process is breaking down food throughout the day and night. Fasting, the process of minimizing or abstaining from food, provides a multitude of benefits to the human body, specifically our digestive tract. But there are other reasons besides weight loss you may choose to fast.

Our intestinal tract, including the small intestine and the large, is approximately fifteen feet in length. How do we care for this amazing and essential part of our inner mechanism?

The physical benefits of fasting range from weight loss and improving cardiovascular health and brain function to reducing blood pressure and inflammation. Individuals on long-term fasts report heightened mental clarity.

Conversely, there are risks. Prolonged fasting may cause dizziness, weakness, nutritional deficiencies, and impact bone health due to reduced intake of calcium and other minerals. It is critical to consult your doctor before beginning any fast.

There are several approaches to fasting, depending on your goal. Since I exercise in the mornings, I usually don't eat until after my workout, which puts me at approximately a sixteen-hour fast daily. Others may argue that breakfast is the most important meal of the day. However, I'm not a morning eater. Coffee, juice, pre-workout drinks, and water keep me going.

Prayer and fasting is common for individuals seeking God's guidance, spiritual strength, empowerment, and intercession, and to break spiritual strongholds. The challenging process of self-discipline and eliminating food is humbling. The main concept for spiritual fasting is that whenever you feel pangs of hunger, it is a reminder to pray.

Intermittent Fasting involves abstaining from eating food for a minimum of twelve hours. Many people already do that from bedtime to breakfast. Or fast for sixteen hours and eat during a six to eight-hour window during the day. This is my preferred method; it gives my digestive system a good break and then I eat after exercising in the morning.

Short-Term Fasting is to forgo food for twenty-four to forty-eight hours.

Extended Fasts are three to forty days. My friend recently fasted for forty days. He kept hydrated by drinking plenty of water, occasionally adding squeezed lemon and honey. He also drank coconut water and herbal tea. Any fast more than three days is very dangerous. The side effects of fasting may include severe headache, inability to fight colds, insomnia, and extreme fatigue. My friend was sick for about a week and I could tell from his voice that his energy was low. He fasted not to lose weight, but to experience what Jesus did. "Then Jesus was led up by the Spirit into the wilderness to be tempted by the devil. And after fasting forty days and forty nights, he was hungry. . . . Then the devil left him, and behold, angels came and were ministering to him," Matthew 4:1–2, 11.

Many Christians observe Lent and fast during the days leading up to Easter. Giving up sugar, sodas, or alcohol is a good place to start. Others find subtle improvements to their overall health and energy by minimizing caloric intake for a day or two once a month.

Whichever way you choose to fast, there are numerous benefits to your body, mind, and spirit. Fasting should be done with caution and understanding the importance of listening to your body. When you fast for any length of time, let someone know your plan. There is no one-size-fits-all approach to fasting, and the benefits may vary based on the type of fasting and duration.

The time between when you take a bite of food until your body has absorbed the nutrition and eliminated the waste can take up to seventy-two hours. Fasting resets this arduous process and leaves you feeling lighter physically and emotionally. Add prayer to fasting as a form of spiritual growth and warfare. Stand your ground and cast out evil forces in the name of Jesus from your life to leave you feeling more at peace, alive, and thriving.

MOVE FORWARD

Except for special occasions, stop eating for the day at 7:00 p.m. From 7:00 p.m. until 7:00 a.m., give your body time to rest from food intake.

PRAYER

Father God, thank you for all the working parts you so intricately made in our bodies. Forgive me for the ways I've neglected my joints and bones and especially my digestive system. I ask for a hedge of protection, Lord, as I approach fasting today. Let me hear your voice, your guidance, and let my body receive greater energy and supernatural health. In Jesus's name, amen.

DAY 10
FORGIVENESS

"Then Peter came up and said to him, 'Lord, how often will my brother sin against me, and I forgive him? As many as seven times?' Jesus said to him, 'I do not say to you seven times, but seventy-seven times.'" Matthew 18:21–22

I pressed my foot on the gas pedal and the engine of my Corvette responded with a deep, guttural thunder. As a former motocross racer, I could handle the extra RPMs. My driving skills were solid, but my emotions were not.

Early Sunday morning, the roads were empty. For a nano second, I wondered what it would be like to drive my car off the upcoming bridge. Would I die on impact with the water? Who would come to my funeral? Would anyone miss me? I considered my five-year-old son, Rocco, and eased up on the pedal. *Yes, someone would miss me.*

Angry, hurt, humiliated, and betrayed, my once purpose-filled life felt shattered. Adultery was not supposed to happen in my marriage. After all, we made promises.

We've all been through emotionally challenging or traumatic situations that cause us to doubt ourselves and doubt our faith. Where is God in our pain?

Times of chronic stress negatively impact our health. My response can vary from over-eating to starving myself because the soul-crushing tragic incident is unbearable. Sleep is impossible. How can I navigate this pain? Will I ever feel peace again? How can I possibly forgive the perpetrator of a heartbreaking offense once, let alone seventy-seven times, as Jesus commanded us?

When all we want to do is scream "it's not fair" or throw a plate at the wall, forgiving is anything but easy. The Lord's prayer encourages us to ask for grace for ourselves and others. We are all flawed. We make mistakes. If God can show mercy when I'm at my worst, then can I do the same and offer forgiveness, grace, and mercy to others? In many cases I question if this is even possible outside of being in relationship with God and His strength. This alone is reason enough to press closer to God.

Lifting weights strengthens muscles. The added pounds and stress of curling dumbbells, leg extensions on a machine, or squats with our own body weight creates tiny tears in our muscle fibers. After a strength-training session, as we allow our bodies to rest, our muscles repair themselves and grow back more powerful. What if we looked at our spiritual bodies in the same way—counting hardships and tribulations as opportunities for growth?

When I look back at difficult times in my life, it's obvious now that they made me more resilient. I'm a different, stronger person today than I was before. However, for years I didn't see past my own dashboard to realize God was moving and growing me in such a beautiful way.

After I nearly died from toxic mold exposure, I spent a year recovering from pre-emphysema and four different types of mold in my bloodstream. I slowly initiated precautions to ensure my home environment remained healthier and free from toxins.

After a devastating betrayal by my husband, I realized the crisis served as an equalizer in my marriage. My opinion mattered. I mattered. I confidently voiced my concerns when previously I had been hesitant. Prior to those two incidents, I operated as a people-pleaser and rolled out the welcome mat for everyone to walk on me. Years later, I unapologetically create boundaries to facilitate my health and happiness.

Like the physical toning I'd put my body through when teaching fitness classes, my discernment became toned. Though I hope I never have to endure that kind of emotional pain again, I learned valuable lessons that I might not have otherwise. I learned I couldn't allow those tribulations to sabotage my physical body and negatively impact my emotional, spiritual, and mental health. Prolonged adversity, anger, and bitterness grow like weeds within the body, choking off joy and wellness. I had to make my emotional and physical health a priority, so I could be of service to others.

A study from the *American Psychological Association* shows that forgiveness of self and others is associated with improved mental and physical health.[*] Increases in forgiveness were associated with decreases in stress and mental health symptoms.

Scripture says it this way: "Get rid of all bitterness, rage and anger, brawling and slander, along with every form of malice. Be kind and compassionate to one another, forgiving each other, just as in Christ God forgave you," Ephesians 4:31–32.

Martin Luther King Jr. said, "We must develop and maintain the capacity to forgive. He who is devoid of the power to forgive is devoid of the power to love." The ultimate example of love and sacrifice is the crucifixion of Jesus. Even when Jesus was on the cross, tortured and dying, his thought was for others. Moments before death, he asked, "Father, forgive them, for they know not what they do," Luke 23:34.

Learning from past mistakes, we forgive ourselves. Challenges make us stronger. When we do the hard work of forgiving others and ourselves, we energize our spiritual capacity and ignite our faith. Like finding a framed family photo in the aftermath of a tornado, forgiveness looks for the good that remains. Releasing the harrowing past, we look toward a new day.

---

[*]   Kirsten Weir, "Forgiveness Can Improve Mental and Physical Health," *Monitor on Psychology*, January 2017, https://www.apa.org/monitor/2017/01/ce-corner.

MOVE FORWARD

What do you need to forgive yourself for? Take the step today to unpack the memory, retain the good lessons learned, and forgive yourself. When this feels hard, remember that God has already forgiven you.

PRAYER

Heavenly Father, I come with a humble heart, grateful for the experiences that have strengthened my mind, body, and soul. Create within me a steadfast longing for you, not only during times of trouble, but through the good times as well. Lord, lift the spirit of heaviness and sadness as described in Isaiah 61:1–3: "He has sent me to bind up the brokenhearted, to proclaim freedom for the captives and release from darkness for the prisoners, to proclaim the year of the Lord's favor and the day of vengeance of our God, to comfort all who mourn, and provide for those who grieve in Zion—to bestow on them a crown of beauty instead of ashes, the oil of joy instead of mourning, and a garment of praise instead of a spirit of despair." In Jesus's mighty name, amen.

WATER: THE FOUNTAIN OF YOUTH

*"But whoever drinks of the water that I will give him will never be thirsty again.
The water that I will give him will become in him a spring of water welling up to eternal life." John 4:14*

On Saturday mornings as a child, I'd eat a bowl of cereal while watching *Scooby Doo* cartoons. Then I'd put on my bathing suit and join my friends at the Clinton River behind my house.

The neighborhood kids and I attached a rope to a beautiful oak tree at the water's edge. All day, we'd swing on the rope and drop into the river. We held swimming and row-boat races, and occasionally went fishing. Even in the murky river, I'd open my eyes underwater. Michigan summers were hot and when we got thirsty, we turned on the spigot behind our house and guzzled water from the hose. I miss those days.

Today, I wouldn't let my dog drink from the river behind my childhood home. On the Michigan Department of Health and Human Services' website, a long list of toxins including mercury, DDT, PCBs, and other cancer-causing chemicals have been found in the Clinton River. The MDHHS warns, "If you are a healthy adult who is not planning on having children in the next several years and you don't fish in an area that has 'Do Not Eat' signs posted by MDHHS, then it is usually okay to eat most Michigan fish one or two times a year."*

Wildlife and marine life need healthy ecosystems without toxic chemicals. Not only is the fish unsafe to eat, swimming in these rivers and lakes can be harmful. Our skin is an organ and absorbs whatever we put on it. Pesticides used in landscaping and agriculture is a prime reason our rivers and lakes are unsafe for swimming or fishing. Billions worldwide suffer from preventable diseases because they don't have access to clean water. Clean water is a necessity for cooking, drinking, and bathing. But where can we get truly pure water?

---

*   Eat Safe Fish FAQs, accessed October 23, 2023, https://www.michigan.gov/mdhhs/-/media/Project /Websites/mdhhs/Folder2/Folder52/Folder1/Folder152/MDCH_EAT_SAFE_FISH_FAQs_WEB .pdf?rev=04a322598eb7429fa38f0ea2591cd67d&hash=B8CB87CD2AA3D7393A937AB7290358D9.

Millions worldwide have turned to drinking water from plastic bottles thinking that's better and safer, but is it? Approximately 60 million plastic water bottles are used each day,[*] most of which wind up in landfills and in the ocean, requiring decades to decompose. Though the use of plastic bottles is commonplace, plastic bottles contain harmful chemicals that leach into the liquid you're drinking. And do you really know the source of the water in that bottle? Some companies use municipal water and use misleading packaging.

Many people use water services that allow them to refill their water jugs. It's less expensive than buying new bottles and you're not contributing to the plastic wasteland in landfills and oceans. We use a whole house water conditioning system that filters many harmful chemicals like PFAs, VOCs, pharmaceutical drugs, and arsenic. The filter adds important minerals like magnesium. The Environmental Working Group provides information about toxic chemicals in the air, soil, and water by zip code.

Human beings need fresh, clean water to survive. H2O is essential for our bodies to function. Dehydration can cause everything from mood swings to kidney stones and urinary tract infections.

How much water is too much? There have been deaths associated with drinking too much water too fast. Water intoxication occurred when a radio contest was held to determine who could drink the most water without using the restroom. Sadly, this contest cost a woman her life.[†]

How much water is the right amount for our bodies and our health? Some say to drink at least half your body weight in ounces of water. I don't adhere to strict guidelines when it comes to how much water to consume and when. Simply put, I listen to my body. When exercising and sweating, I drink more water than when I'm sitting at a desk, writing. I try not to drink liquids an hour or two before bed to minimize bathroom trips in the middle of the night. In higher elevations, when I'm skiing, I am extra cautious to hydrate more than normal.

Symptoms of dehydration include:

- Brain fog
- Dark urine
- Dizziness
- Dry mouth/thirst
- Headache
- Lethargy
- Sore throat

---

[*]   Joey, "74 Shocking Plastic Water Bottle Pollution Facts & Statistics (2023)," Jersey Island Holidays, May 26, 2023, https://www.jerseyislandholidays.com/plastic-bottle-pollution-statistics/#chapter-2.

[†]   "Woman Dies after Water-Drinking Contest," NBCNews.com, January 14, 2007, https://www.nbcnews.com/id/wbna16614865.

Toxic chemicals that could be in your municipal water include:

- Ammonia
- Chromium
- Cyanide
- Fluoride
- Lead
- Pesticides
- Pharmaceutical drugs
- PFAs & PFOs
- Sulfates
- Volatile Organic Compounds

STAY HYDRATED

Tips and ideas to help you get and stay hydrated include:

- Infuse water with fruits and veggies
- Drink spring water or filtered water from reverse osmosis
- Set hourly reminders on your phone
- On glass mason jars write 1, 2, 3 . . . to monitor your progress of consumption
- Drink one full glass of water as soon as you wake up, and one glass before each meal
- Add hydration sticks to water
- Track your water intake daily, consuming at least five 8-ounce glasses of water per day

MOVE FORWARD

Check with your doctor to determine exactly how much water you should drink and when. Those with illnesses including diabetes are at greater risk for dehydration. Do your research to find a beneficial water filtration system. (See Resources, page 161.)

PRAYER

Father, thank you for the amazing gift of water and its benefits. Help me appreciate this blessing and freely and abundantly help others who are struggling to have something as simple as clean water. Protect the rivers and lakes from spoiling and poisoning. Let us all have the bounty of precious, life-giving water. Please provide an abundance of health and hydration so I can continue to do your good work. In Jesus's name, amen.

DAY 12
CRAVINGS

"Be not among drunkards
or among gluttonous eaters of meat,
for the drunkard and the glutton will come to poverty,
and slumber will clothe them with rags."
Proverbs 23:20–21

Does your mind work like mine? My mind can trick me into believing I need something that I really don't. Oftentimes, I can be duped into thinking that one particular food I've enjoyed in the past will reward me with feelings of delight and satisfaction. These thoughts are strongest when I'm fatigued, overwhelmed, stressed, or brokenhearted. Hard day at work? Eat a cookie and experience a moment of sweet bliss.

After getting the quick mood boost, my thoughts plunge me into disappointment in myself. How could I have given in and eaten something I know is not beneficial for my body? How could I have betrayed my resolution to be mindful of my diet?

But food addictions and cravings aren't entirely our fault. Dopamine levels in our brain regulate the pleasure/pain/reward centers and spike whenever we eat or drink something that appealed previously. Food manufacturers spend millions of dollars in advertisements and packaging that send our sensory perception into overdrive and tantalize the taste buds.

Yes, we may feel a momentary rush of energy watching a celebrity, or perfectly coiffed spokesperson, touting a drink or snack. Sugar, salt, fat, and flavor enhancers are added to foods many people consume daily including milk, bread, and packaged foods, making it difficult to consume less. Sugar is added to a vast array of foods. Because sugar is as addictive as cocaine, the consumer is drawn back again and again in impulse buys.[*] We crave what is not good for us.

Cravings and addictions can be a way to cope with stressful situations, or simply become long-term habits that are difficult to break. Every time you sit down to watch television, do you feel the urge to have chips or a snack? Although you may feel full after a meal, are you

---

[*] David J Mysels and Maria A Sullivan, "The Relationship between Opioid and Sugar Intake: Review of Evidence and Clinical Applications," *Journal of Opioid Management*, 2010, https://www.ncbi.nlm.nih.gov/pmc/articles/PMC3109725/.

tempted to have just one bite of pie? Are you prompted at parties to taste an appetizer even when you're not hungry?

The media influences us subliminally. In the movie *When Harry Met Sally*, Meg Ryan's character fakes an orgasm in a restaurant. Another patron watching the actress's hilarious but convincing demonstration says to her waitress, "I'll have what she's having." Psychologically, if others look successful, content, or deliriously happy with a particular food or drink, we reason that perhaps that is the thing that will provide what we are missing.

Our neurotransmitters can be deceiving. Ice cream, while cold and very enjoyable on a hot summer day, will probably not save us from heat stroke—unless it's the only thing to eat.

Cravings can also be caused by nutritional and hormonal imbalances. Magnesium, vitamin B, and zinc deficiencies may cause cravings for chocolate, sweets, and even red meat. The hormones leptin and ghrelin signal fullness after a meal. A deficiency in these hormones can also contribute to food cravings.[*] Check with your doctor to discover more about why your body craves certain foods. A few tweaks may help control unhealthy urges to snack, binge, and overindulge.

CURB CRAVINGS

Rewiring our brain circuitry with a few tricks can help curb our cravings.

- List the times/days/activities when you indulge in food or drink that are unhealthy
- Create a list of healthy snacks you can swap
- Manage stress
- Exercise daily
- Drink more water
- Phone a friend and share your experiences
- Eat well-balanced meals
- Consume enough protein
- Get adequate sleep
- Eat more fiber
- Pray before you eat
- Keep a food journal
- Avoid white sugar and white flour
- Cut back where you can. For example, eliminate whipped cream on top of your sugary iced mocha, and request half the amount of syrup.
- Don't bring it home. If you buy junk food, you're more apt to consume it.

---

[*] Alina Petre, "What Do Food Cravings Mean? Facts and Myths, Explained," *Healthline*, July 20, 2023, https://www.healthline.com/nutrition/craving-meanings#causes.

- Chew slowly and breathe
- Become a label reader and minimize packaged food with added sugar and man-made chemicals
- Minimize snacks with empty calories

Occasionally we want to enjoy the cake a friend baked for our birthday, or the cookies a grandchild brought over, and that's ok. It's also ok to take a day off from exercising occasionally. When 80 percent of your diet is healthy, you can reset your psyche to get back on track to healthier living after the party is over. Here are three steps to get motivated.

1. **Exercise longer, not harder.** If you work out too hard, too fast, you are more prone to injuries, which cause more delays. Instead, increase the duration and work out at a moderate pace to burn calories and get back on track to healthy living. If you like to walk, merely walk longer at the same pace.
2. **Go cold turkey.** Decide ahead of time to say no to junk food. The sooner you can pass up the cake, cookies, and potato chips, the better. Fill up on meat, salads, and vegetables. Don't purchase unhealthy items. If it's not in the house, you won't be tempted.
3. **Call a friend.** Motivation comes when you make a date with a friend to go to a gym, take a walk, or at least check in on each other to see how you're doing. Accountability is key to staying on track. Plan your workouts and write them into your schedule just like an important meeting. We often put others before ourselves, but after indulging, it's time to make your health a priority.

MOVE FORWARD

What one thing from the list above will you begin today?

PRAYER

Heavenly Father, I thank you for this day. When many around the world are starving, we are blessed to live in a country where food is plentiful. Help me honor my sacred temple, this body, with nourishing meat, fish, and vegetables that you designed. Father, I struggle with food cravings and addictions. I humbly ask for your grace. Help me avoid junk food and empty calories that do not energize my body. I can do all things through you who gives me strength (Philippians 4:13). Help me to make healthy food choices. In Jesus's name, amen.

THREE ELEMENTS TO EXERCISE

"She dresses herself with strength and makes her arms strong." Proverbs 31:17

Sherry never missed my Zumba class, and I admired her dedication. She stayed after our sixty minutes of high-intensity dance-inspired workouts to take a strength-training or yoga class. Retired, Sherry seemed happy, devoting time to exercise every day.

Secretly, I felt envious. With a teenage son in school, a husband who traveled for work, and several businesses to oversee, I barely had three hours a week to teach my fitness classes, never mind to do extra workouts.

Invited to speak at the American Heart Association's Go Red for Women luncheon, I was surprised to see Sherry. "What are you doing here?"

She opened the top of her blouse revealing the scar from open heart surgery when she was in her forties. Like others who have experienced life-threatening wake-up calls, Sherry realized the importance of prioritizing health and balancing three essential components: work, family, and rest.

Life is a juggling act to balance your job, homelife, parenting, chores, charity, and more. We often don't devote enough time to managing the stress that comes with these daily obligations until it's too late. We might feel we're getting enough exercise walking the dog, but there are several important elements for a complete workout: Cardio, strength training, and stretching.

EXERCISE BASICS

While cardiovascular exercises like dancing, brisk walking, and swimming lower the risk of heart disease and stroke, weight training and stretching are key to overall health and wellness, especially as we age. As decades pass, we lose bone density and joint mobility, which contributes to fractures when senior citizens reach their seventies, eighties, and nineties. Stretching also prevents injuries.

A study from the Centers for Disease Control and Prevention concluded that in 2020, only 21 percent of adults between the ages of fifty and sixty-four met the basic physical activity guidelines. That number decreased to 15 percent for seniors over sixty-five.[*]

Sherry's winning combination incorporated cardiovascular exercise, which lowers the risk of heart disease, with strength training and stretching. The three elements of cardio, strength training, and stretching provides a well-rounded, safe, and effective workout that prevents injuries, develops muscle, and increases bone density.

Here's a sample of my favorite thirty-minute workout:

1. **Warm-up (5 minutes):** Warming up the body prepares muscles and joints for the work ahead by getting blood flowing throughout the body. Start with small movements that gradually become larger. For example: shoulder rolls before arm circles that reach high and increase your range of motion. Think of taffy for a moment. When it's cold, taffy is brittle and breaks. Warm taffy is soft and pliable. The same is true for muscles. Save longer stretching for after the workout. Gentle movement that twists the torso and elongates the spine, arms, and legs are optimum for warm-ups.

2. **Cardio (10 minutes):** Dancing, cycling, swimming, running, or other aerobic activities that get your heart rate elevated between 50 to 85 percent of your maximum heart rate (MHR) is preferred. Check with your doctor to determine your MHR and how often and how long you should exercise each week. Drugs like beta blockers may prevent an elevated heart rate.[†]

3. **Strength Training (10 minutes):** Use your own bodyweight, dumbbells, machines, or bands that cause resistance within a muscle group. Two or three sets of eight to twelve repetitions are optimal. If you easily reach twelve reps and don't feel challenged, increase the weight. There is a fine line between pushing yourself and getting injured. Consult a trainer to help you get started. Make sure you rest the muscle group you're targeting for at least thirty-six hours. The recovery time allows the muscle to become stronger.

4. **Cool Down (5 minutes):** This is absolutely my favorite part of the workout. Elevating heart rate and toning muscles releases feel-good hormones. Breathe deeply and hold stretches for a minimum of thirty seconds each. Think of elongating your neck, torso, arms, and legs. Lie flat on the floor, take one bent knee across your body,

---

[*] "Physical Activity Among Adults Aged 18 and Over: United States, 2020," Centers for Disease Control and Prevention, August 30, 2022, https://www.cdc.gov/nchs/products/databriefs/db443.htm#section_1.

[†] "Target Heart Rate for Exercise," University of Iowa Hospitals & Clinics, accessed October 24, 2023, https://uihc.org/health-topics/target-heart-rate-exercise.

twisting and stretching your low back. Repeat on the other side. The yoga move downward dog is an excellent full body stretch.

MOVE FORWARD

As bodies in motion, when we're stressed, we forget that stillness and stretching are incredible gifts. After your next workout, give yourself the gift of rest and relaxation.

PRAYER

Heavenly Father, my heart is full of gratitude for strength in my muscles and bones, and for joints that are flexible. Every day, I am amazed at your creation and the opportunities I have to get stronger and healthier. You created my heart, lungs, and organs to function. Help me find time to make exercise a part of my daily life so that I can be abundantly well. In Jesus's name, amen.

DAY 14
DETOXIFY YOUR HOME

"By wisdom a house is built, and by understanding it is established; by knowledge the rooms are filled with all precious and pleasant riches." Proverbs 24:3-4

The first time I met with the doctor at the Environmental Health Center in Dallas, I reached for the water bottle in my purse. The doctor shook his head. "You can't drink out of plastic ever again."

Learning about chemicals in plastic bottles that leach into the liquid was the beginning of my education in environmental toxins. As part of my healing process, I lived near the clinic in an apartment carefully prepared for chemically-sensitive and chemically-overloaded patients. This living space held no carpeting, no toxic cleaning chemicals, no potpourri, scented candles, or scented trash bags. The apartment did smell like snickerdoodle cookies from the Austin air purifier that cleaned the air of dust and other potential contaminants.

Within the facility many common household products were banned including hair spray, nail polish, perfume, and clothes washed in chemically scented soaps and dried with fabric softeners. People like me who were sick and couldn't get answers from other doctors came from around the globe to be treated by Dr. William Rea in a desperate search to feel better.

At Dr. Rea's Environmental Health Center there were treatment rooms for detoxifying therapies like infrared saunas, vitamin IVs, and allergy testing. Inside one particular room separated by a glass wall were a dozen people receiving IV treatments. I asked the woman sitting next to me, "What's that room for?"

"That's for the really sick people who are allergic to everything," she explained. "They can't wear leather belts or shoes because those are chemically treated and off-gas, leaching noxious chemicals in the air. They can't bring in newspapers, books, or magazines because the ink on the paper is toxic."

Suddenly I felt like one of the lucky ones as I considered their challenges.

Back home, I quickly realized that I will always be sensitive to chemical additives like the fragrance plug-ins, scented candles, and fabric softener. That fake "fresh clean scent" can cause headaches, weight gain, and possibly even cancer. I learned to shop for natural cleaners and to make my own.

While undergoing treatment with Dr. Rea, I couldn't attend the first parent-teacher conference at my son's new school. Although Dr. Rea wanted me to stay three months, I missed my family and returned home after four weeks. I was weak, but alive. Like a non-smoker can recognize a smoker from the lingering scent of tobacco, my sense of smell was heightened by every little thing. When I entered Rocco's new school, I instantly felt like I was hit by a Mack truck of noxious air. The school's gym floor had recently been resurfaced and the deadly chemical scent instantly triggered a debilitating headache. Fortunately, the teachers were receptive to my predicament and agreed to meet with me outside the school.

Dodging debilitating smells endured. When I filled my gas tank, the fuel fumes zapped my energy for hours. It was months before I could go into a mall or restaurant without becoming ill.

WHAT TO ELIMINATE

While a controversial topic among physicians, Multiple Chemical Sensitivity (MCS) is a very real diagnosis for my family and millions of others. Like a canary in a coal mine, I can walk into a freshly painted space and tell if the paint was regular VOC paint, low-VOC, or no VOC. Paints with volatile organic compounds (VOCs) trigger flu-like symptoms, allergies and more. Oftentimes, I can sense if there's mildew or toxic mold.

Chemically scented candles give headaches. That new car smell is actually the off-gassing of formaldehyde and other toxic chemicals used to treat materials for the carpet, dashboards, and seat covers. Removing all poisonous toxins from your world is impossible. Even if you ate only organic food from your garden, you're still exposed to air pollution, chlorofluorocarbon, vehicle emissions, pesticides, fireproofing, heavy metals, soil contamination, electromagnetic pollution, volatile organic compounds, radiation, volcanic ash, bacteria, pollen, and parasites. Some health organizations estimate that exposure to environmental pollutants cause 25 percent of all deaths and diseases globally.[*]

Harmful toxins in our air, soil, and water contribute to the toxic load in our bodies. The higher the toxic load and the more poisons we ingest, the more difficult it is to feel well. A runny nose might be caused by pollution, pollen, chemicals, or toxic mold.

Whether chemically sensitive or not, become aware of hazardous chemicals in products you consume. Trash bags, tissues, laundry soap, fabric softener, air fresheners, and colorful candles claim to provide a fresh clean scent. Actually, they mask odors, increase the toxins in the air, and contribute to upper respiratory symptoms including headaches, runny nose, watery eyes, brain fog, coughing, sore throat, and breathing trouble. Read labels and research the ingredients in products you use.

Most laundry detergent, fabric softener, and dryer sheets contain chemical scents that lead to a night of tossing and turning, and potential serious health conditions. That naturally

---

[*] "Ambient (Outdoor) Air Pollution," World Health Organization, accessed October 24, 2023, https://www.who.int/news-room/fact-sheets/detail/ambient-(outdoor)-air-quality-and-health.

fresh scent listed on a plastic jug of laundry soap comes from harsh chemicals, not nature. Manufacturers use natural sounding phrases like "clean burst," "spring scent," and "mountain fresh" to sound like we're buying something healthy. Who doesn't love the pretty lavender flowers on containers?

Ever wonder why ingredients aren't listed on laundry soap packaging? There's no law requiring the manufacturers to disclose how they get that phony mountain fresh, springtime flowery fragrance. Synthetic ingredients like sodium lauryl sulfate and nonylphenol ethoxylate can cause skin rashes, organ toxicity, low sperm count, reproductive issues, hormone disruption, and cancer. If it's in your laundry detergent or dryer sheets, that means the chemicals are on your skin and in the air.

Perhaps you still don't want to give up your spring-meadow-clean-burst laundry soap or fabric softener. Since you are not experiencing symptoms *now*, you might not think the product is harmful to your family or pets. However, what are these chemicals doing to the environment? Those harmful substances are released into the air, soil, and water, polluting wildlife habitat and contributing to ozone depletion. If you want to save the environment, eliminate the use of chemically scented laundry soaps and fabric softeners.

Check the labels of cleaning products in your home and research the side effects of these ingredients.

MOVE FORWARD

What products can you remove from your home this week to create a healthier environment?

PRAYER

Dear God, thank you for the beautiful world you created for us to live in. Give me wisdom and discernment to know what is good for me and those in my circle of influence. Make me aware of unhealthy products to eliminate to make a health-supporting environment. In Jesus's name, amen.

FIVE STEPS TO WEIGHT LOSS & MAINTENANCE

"Not that I am speaking of being in need, for I have learned in whatever situation I am to be content. I know how to be brought low, and I know how to abound. In any and every circumstance, I have learned the secret of facing plenty and hunger, abundance and need. I can do all things through him who strengthens me." Philippians 4:12–13

"Is that me?"

My eyesight has become worse the past few years, so when I looked behind me in the fitting room mirror, I wondered if the image was just blurry.

Those are definitely not my legs.

The legs reflected in the mirror were dimpled with cottage cheese–like cellulite, saggy, and far from muscular.

The mirror must be wrong. I've worked out all my life. How could it be that I missed how unattractive the backs of my legs had become? Looking closer, I realized the reflected image showed my untoned, out of shape backside in the mirror. God bless my husband for all the times when he said my body was a "wonderland" and beautiful. Maybe he needed glasses, too.

For women over fifty, maintaining or losing weight can sometimes feel like an uphill battle. It has been for me. The strategies I used when I was younger, even at age forty, don't work anymore. Hormones are changing, I'm much less active, and I'm losing muscle tone and elasticity in my joints.

Here is the plan I'm doing to get back in shape and maintain my weight:

1. Pick a number. Pick a reasonable and attainable target weight and measurement for your waist and hips. Stay within ten pounds of your target weight. Your waist to hip (WHR) ratio often determines a predisposition for diabetes and even early death.[*]
2. Step it up a notch. Exercise is one of the most important things you can do for your overall health. Movement improves mood, boosts energy, and lowers risk of chronic

---

[*] "Waist to Hip Ratio Calculator," https://www.omnicalculator.com/health/waist-hip-ratio.

disease. Include a mix of strength training, cardio, and stretching in your routine. If you're serious about toning and weight loss, increase the intensity, frequency, and/or the duration of your workouts. To increase the intensity, lift heavier weights, jump higher, and walk faster. Visualize your muscles contracting as you engage in strength training. Exercise longer—instead of thirty minutes, go for sixty. Make your workouts more frequent.

3. Food swap. Switch processed and sugary foods for whole foods. Processed foods are typically loaded with additives and preservatives. Instead, opt for whole foods like garden fresh fruits and vegetables, venison, chicken, and meat from local farmers. These foods are packed with nutrients and help you feel your best (see Day 30).

4. Avoid late night snacking. Late night eating increases risk for heart disease, diabetes, and causes sleep disruptions and weight gain.

5. Manage stress. Stress can have a negative impact on your health, so it's important to find ways to manage it. Meditation and prayer are ways to relax and reduce stress, especially before bed. Stress hormones like cortisol send your body into the fight or flight mode, which is good if you're fighting a tiger, but not so good on a daily basis. After the adrenaline surges in your body, you burn muscle rather than fat, and you'll probably be hungrier. While our bodies adapt to physical and mental stress, we also need periods of rest and recuperation. Walk outside, close your eyes, and breathe deeply. Listen to the birds, feel the wind, and visualize your body relaxing.

MOVE FORWARD

What is your target weight and the number you will not allow yourself to weigh more than? Which days of the week will you exercise? Which foods can you commit to swapping? Instead of late night snacking, try a gentle nighttime stretch.

PRAYER

Heavenly Father, I am filled with gratitude for this body you've sculpted, a wondrous creation that moves, feels, and breathes. In every step I take, every gesture I make, I want to glorify you and honor this temple you've entrusted to me—cellulite, saggy skin, and all. Fill me with unwavering strength, immeasurable discipline, and an outpouring of energy and stamina to follow through with this 40-Day Abundantly Well journey. I can do all things through you: I can lose weight and tone my muscles. In Jesus's name, amen.

DAY 16
PRAYER & MEDITATION

"Be still, and know that I am God." Psalm 46:10

Two weeks after receiving a contract to write this book, *Abundantly Well*, I felt incredibly *unwell*. In fact, I felt like I was dying. How could I proclaim that I knew how to get abundantly healthier and happier when I pulled a muscle in my back, I couldn't eat or sleep, and my dog was dying?

Barely functioning in my zombie state, I made a commitment to write about overcoming obstacles, finding joy, and supernatural health.

A few years ago, when I felt more like a teenage gymnast than fifty-five, I could leap into a split jump, do a cartwheel, followed by the splits. But now, in the arctic air-conditioned waiting room at Texas A&M Small Animal Veterinary Hospital, I sat hunched over, head in my hands, as a tear dropped on the tile floor. *Don't cry, don't cry, don't cry.*

I texted a few friends. "Please pray for Happy. They think it could be cancer." My husband, Ted, and I have an unhealthy attachment to our dogs. On his farewell tour, Ted chartered a plane and flew home to see his best friend in the world, our dog Happy. *One more time.*

I had a lot of time to contemplate the fragility of life during the 220-mile round-trip I took five times in two weeks to Texas A&M veterinary hospital. As Happy teetered on life support, I needed to overcome the anxiety and stress. I couldn't care for Happy if I wasn't healthy.

On the second day at A&M, Happy had a seizure. On the third day, they asked me not to visit so he wouldn't expend precious energy getting excited. His heart was failing and his lungs were peppered with black spots. I prayed during those hours on the road. I thanked God for the wonderful years we'd already had with our pup. *Could there be more days?*

On the fourth day, I met with the veterinarian. *Was she smiling?*

"We've never seen anything like this." The veterinarian said that in four days, Happy's x-rays were 70 percent clearer. The mass on his heart was gone.

While Happy was not fully recovered, it's hard to see this drastic improvement any other way than a miracle. Most of us are aware of the potent power of faith and prayer. What if we prayed and surrendered all our troubles to God? I know, easier said than done.

When faced with a challenge, I begin with baby steps.

P. R.A.Y.

Find a purposeful way to pray that works for you. The P. R.A.Y. acronym is an easy system. See if it works for you.

P—Praise God and his glorious works. From the birds chirping, the smell of basil, a smiling baby, and the feel of your pet's fur as you snuggle, find things for which you're grateful.

R—Repent of your sins. Ask forgiveness for the errors you've willingly and unwillingly been a part of.

A—Ask God for guidance, healing, and comfort. Bring your personal petitions to him.

Y—Yield to the opportunities God places before you. Trust him.

PRAYER FOR STRENGTH

Heavenly Father, I come humbly, and with gratitude. Thank you for healing me in troubling times. When I couldn't see it immediately, you answered my prayers in ways I never thought possible. Forgive me for my transgressions, they are many. I repent of sins I knowingly or unknowingly participated in. You have given authority to walk on snakes and scorpions and overcome all the power of the enemy according to Luke 10:19. I ask for a hedge of protection around my home, family, and pets. In Jesus's mighty name, amen.

Here are Scripture passages to encourage your heart.

"Do not be anxious about anything, but in everything by prayer and supplication with thanksgiving let your requests be made known to God. And the peace of God, which surpasses all understanding, will guard your hearts and your minds in Christ Jesus," comforts Philippians 4:6–7.

"Therefore I tell you, whatever you ask in prayer, believe that you have received it, and it will be yours," says Mark 11:24.

"Behold, I have given you authority to tread on serpents and scorpions, and over all the power of the enemy, and nothing shall hurt you," assures Luke 10:19.

MEDITATION AND PRAYER TIPS

Establishing a consistent routine that includes prayer and meditation can lower blood pressure, relieve stress, and improve overall health.

Set the timer for a minimum of three minutes.

Find a relaxing place to sit.

Close your eyes and take several deep breaths.

As you exhale, notice stress, pain, and negativity reduce in your body and mind.

Keep taking large breaths of air in through your nose and allow the exhaled air to slowly release through your mouth, making an O shape with your lips.

Do a mental body scan and recognize the areas where you hold tension. Your neck, jaw, back, and stomach can be containers for anxiety.

Envision your cells getting stronger and happier. Believe that energy courses through your veins.

Allow a smile, however slight, to come to your face.

Remain for a while to allow yourself to feel serenity.

What limiting beliefs or patterns hold you back?

How can you redefine your habits and thoughts?

What negative thoughts come up for you? How do they make you feel, and what positive affirmations can you use to replace them?

Talk to the Lord and allow yourself the quiet waiting to hear God speak to you.

Afterwards, think back to your prayer and meditation experience.

Where did you feel tension in your body?

Did you feel lighter, less pain, or a bit happier?

What was the best part of your experience?

With daily prayer and meditation practice, you change your outlook on life, even during difficult times. Picture your body getting stronger and healthier and your mind will move toward making your vision become reality.

MOVE FORWARD

Think of a situation that's troubling you right now. Ask God to heal your anxious heart. Take a walk outside, make a cup of tea, and meditate on calming your accelerating pulse. Health multiplies as we experience God's peace.

PRAYER

Father, it's difficult sometimes to ignore the chaos and hardship in this world. I become sad and overwhelmed sometimes. Help me slow down and move with intention. Fill my heart with peace today. In Jesus's name, amen.

DAY 17
HORMONAL HAVOC

"For God gave us a spirit not of fear
but of power and love and self-control." 2 Timothy 1:7

I seriously thought I was immune to it. After being a fitness professional and healthy lifestyle guru for decades, when others proclaimed the angst they had about belly fat or profuse sweating caused by menopause, I thought I had dodged a bullet. A hysterectomy in my forties put me in the menopause club a little early. After fully healing, I resumed teaching high intensity fitness classes several times a week and felt great.

One day, without any warning, symptoms hit like a thunderbolt and I knew exactly what it was. I was in a meeting in a swanky restaurant wearing a beautiful light blue dress when suddenly I felt like someone dropped a bucket of water on me. Sweat spewed from every pore in my body. Not only uncomfortable, the situation was also embarrassing. My beautiful blue dress was sweat-stained and ruined. I had not escaped the torture of menopause.

After women have experienced painful menstrual cycles and the agony of childbirth, with menopause comes a whole new set of aches and pains. Additionally, as we age, our hormone levels change causing weight gain, hot flashes, insomnia, headaches, vaginal dryness, fatigue and, as if that wasn't enough, we're pretty darn moody at times.

While I recognize the need for western medicine and have relied on it at times throughout my life, I don't subscribe to hormone replacement therapy in the usual definition. I tried several approaches, but the side effects were disproportionate to the payoff. Instead, I manage the hormonal roller-coaster ride with a ketogenic diet, supplements, and exercise, along with prayer and meditation.

Symptoms are different for every woman. Some experience symptoms that are extraordinarily severe. Consult a trusted gynecologist to help ascertain the best menopause treatment for you and your lifestyle.

NATURAL REMEDIES

- Exercise daily to soothe the effects of water retention and to boost your mood.
- Manage stress with laughter, meditation, and prayer.

- Many women find success alleviating their symptoms with the herbal or vitamin supplements such as black cohosh, soy isoflavones, flaxseed, evening primrose oil, red clover, vitamin D, and calcium.
- Start slowly. Try one supplement for a week, then add another the following week. With this pace, you'll be able to better determine how each affects your physical symptoms.
- Take a probiotic to maintain healthy bacteria in your digestive tract.
- Stay hydrated.
- Give yourself grace. There is no magic pill or textbook cure that works for everyone. We don't always get it right the first time. We are perfectly human. We spill milk. The quicker we clean it up, the quicker we move on to the next right thing.
- Get a blood test to monitor hormones progesterone, estrogen, and testosterone, as well as magnesium and inflammation in your body.

The unspoken truth about menopause is that we've reached the second half of our lives, and that can be depressing. We are no longer childbearing age. Our skin sags and bruises more easily. Our muscle tone isn't what it once was. Miniskirts are out of the question. With our children grown, we are alone more often. Are we attractive or desirable?

The good news is that if we embrace these changes and do what we can holistically, we can *and will* manage the symptoms. We can use this phase of our lives as a reawakening. No more tampons! We may have more free time to do the things we once dreamed of. Start a new business, read more, or take a cooking class. At one time, having lunch with a friend might have seemed like a luxury. Recultivate cherished friendships and focus on the things that matter most. Reimagine how you'd like the second half of your life to be.

For women, menopause is a natural part of aging that we shouldn't fear, although unexpected hot flashes can feel overwhelming. My husband knows not to argue with me when we're driving in the car and I suddenly blast the air conditioning on my face. Smart guy. Aging with grace is showing the world we've worked hard, experienced devastating loss, incredible joy, and have the wrinkles and gray hairs to prove it.

MOVE FORWARD

What exciting new activity can you incorporate into your life? Schedule one today.

PRAYER

Father God, I am here, humbled and overjoyed to have reached this amazing time in life. Help me remember to give myself grace and not to relish my embarrassing mishaps. You have given me a powerful spirit and sound mind. Let me use them to honor you, Father, in all that I do. I love you. In Jesus's mighty name, amen.

DAY 18
MIND MANAGEMENT

"Do not be conformed to this world, but be transformed by the renewal of your mind, that by testing you may discern what is the will of God, what is good and acceptable and perfect." Romans 12:2

In the movie *Dumb and Dumber*, actor Jim Carrey asks his love interest if there is a chance she'd consider dating him. The odds of the two of them getting together, the actress replies, are "About one in a million."

Jim Carrey reacts with a sly grin. "So you're saying there's a chance."

Similarly, having a spirit-filled, positive mindset can give us hope. Maybe you've tried dozens of diets and exercise routines and may have had some success, but not enough to make a difference. When situations in our lives don't turn out as we expect or when we think we cannot change bad luck, we can spiral into perpetual feelings of frustration and fear. When we make a decision to give up or focus on the frustration that something isn't working the way we hoped, a chemical reaction in our brain switches off the feel-good hormone oxytocin. Subconsciously, we give ourselves permission to fail.

So, how do you get motivated to make changes and stay upbeat and positive regardless of a potentially negative outcome? What if you reimagined the possibilities for your life, redefined new truths, and reframed your approach to living fully and aging gracefully?

You can retrain your brain with neuroplasticity, prayer, and deliverance. Transformation comes from the renewing of your mind. A study from the University of Colorado Boulder found that positive belief, especially the deep-seated kind, dramatically affects stress levels and mental health.

Moving past frustration and into a positive outlook begins with our mind. The Bible gives the key: "Finally, brothers, whatever is true, whatever is honorable, whatever is just, whatever is pure, whatever is lovely, whatever is commendable, if there is any excellence, if there is anything worthy of praise, think about these things," Philippians 4:8.

We cannot keep thoughts from coming to mind, but we do control how long they remain. As each criticism comes, mentally say, "Yes, and," putting in a positive note. When you criticize, complain, condemn, or make excuses about your health, quickly remind yourself, "Yes, and I'm bravely on the path to make improvements."

The American Psychological Association suggests that focusing on positives and building resilience can lead to reduced stress and better mental health.[*] Whenever I get stuck in stinking thinking and allow previous failures to hijack my thoughts, I consider how I can renew my mind. Redefining a new truth may give you a renewed mindset.

When you first tried to ride a bicycle or tie your shoes, most likely you took a spill or got frustrated with the laces. But you kept trying until you achieved a fair amount of success. Like many things we attempt in life, whether it's skiing, golfing, or cooking, we usually have to be persistent until we accomplish an acceptable level of competency. Can you give yourself some grace, curiosity, and childlike excitement? Something as simple as trying a different recipe in the kitchen of life may be just what the doctor ordered.

The truth is that with every breath you take, you have an opportunity to rise above the ominous clouds that have suppressed your light for far too long. You're tired, God knows, but if you give up now, hang up your dancing shoes, you'll never realize the incredible joy God has in store. Grab the popcorn! The best part of the movie is about to begin: the rest of your life *on God's terms.*

Every time you say something negative about someone, including yourself, you decrease your body's ability to function at its peak. With your own negative thoughts and words, you suppress your immune system. Toxic thinking can increase your blood pressure and lead to a variety of serious health issues. If you do not see yourself as God sees you, read through the Bible and highlight every verse that tells how God feels about you. In his eyes, you are beautiful, amazing, and talented. "Do not let your adorning be external—the braiding of hair and the putting on of gold jewelry, or the clothing you wear—but let your adorning be the hidden person of the heart with the imperishable beauty of a gentle and quiet spirit, which in God's sight is very precious," 1 Peter 3:3–4. Whenever you doubt your worth, search God's Word for the truth and root out lies that might be holding you back.

You've experienced bleak times and soul-stirring wounds, but God's grace is infused in your body, mind, and soul. Maybe you forgot about the activities you did as a child that brought you joy. Maybe you lost sight of who you really are at your core. Ask God to help you remember and reawaken that inner spark of joy despite the betrayals and tribulations.

MOVE FORWARD

For one full day, each time your thoughts turn to negativity, shift to positive. Notice how different you feel at the end of the day. The next day, repeat.

---

[*] "Building Your Resilience," American Psychological Association, accessed October 25, 2023, https://www.apa.org/topics/resilience/building-your-resilience.

PRAYER

Father, my heart is overflowing with appreciation that you sent your only son to die for me. As I walk through the day and sleep at night, reveal your instructions to live a more holy life. Search my heart and remove the toxic thinking that troubles me. I trust that you are guiding my steps for your purpose. You are with me always and I love you. In Jesus's name, amen.

RELIEVE ACHES & PAINS

"The Lord is my rock and my fortress and my deliverer,
my God, my rock, in whom I take refuge,
my shield, and the horn of my salvation, my stronghold." Psalm 18:2

When my husband, Ted, had both of his knees replaced, he was in an incredible amount of agony, even with anesthesia. I tried something with him that I knew had helped me with debilitating migraines. While the technique won't completely take away the pain of a critical injury, this eased the stress for Ted.

Meditation, relaxation, and finding distractions from overwhelmingly negative thoughts is proven to relieve stress and pain during difficult times. I invited Ted to close his eyes.

"Picture what that pain looks like in your mind's eye." After a pause, I continued, "Give the pain a shape, a color—something dark—and even a name. What does it look like?"

He nodded when he was there.

"Now, take several long, deep breaths," I coached. "With your eyes still closed, picture the air coming into your lungs as a bright color. Watch it spread throughout your body. Soon, your body becomes a brighter, healthier, more vivacious color that now takes over the pain. Watch as the dark color and shape of the thing you called pain is exhaled."

After several minutes, Ted visibly felt more at ease.

Part of being healthy and happy is not only based upon what we eat and how we exercise, but how we think and feel. Scientists are discovering links between our emotions and our health. Think of couples who have been together for a long time and when one dies the other soon follows although they had no terminal health problems. Grief can have an astonishing effect on the human body and cause heart attacks and strokes.

BODY SOUNDS

It started with the typical symptoms of sneezing, stuffy nose, runny nose, headache, and fatigue, but I was too busy to listen to my body. I had been doing interviews to promote my new book, *4 Minutes a Day, Rock 'n' Roll Your Way to Happy*, producing our TV show, *Ted*

Nugent Spirit of the Wild, and keeping up on chores like cooking, cleaning, laundry, and paying bills. In several interviews, I even bragged that "I never get sick."

At last, I was diagnosed with a sinus infection. The lesson I learned is to listen to my body. Sometimes aches and pains come because we worked out hard and our muscles were pushed to their limit and beyond. Other times, we experience aches and pains because our body is telling us we are sick and need recovery.

Listen to the signals your body gives. For sore muscles, the best response is the R.I.C.E. method. Rest, Ice, Compression, Elevation. In the case of illness or injury, your body may require extra attention to return to good health. If you are not sure what your body is telling you, get an opinion from a trusted professional in healthcare. If your gut does not agree with a diagnosis, get a second opinion. Often a chiropractor can adjust tendons, muscles, and skeletal alignments, a doctor can run blood tests, a functional doctor can look deeper into a problem, and a naturopath can suggest a healing path.

In the case of illness:

1. **It's okay to rest.** Sometimes you have to put your life on pause. Being stressed and overworked is a laboratory for illness. Give yourself permission to have downtime without the guilt. Sleep as much as you can as healing is multiplied when we sleep.
2. **Cold plunge.** While the temperature of water can vary, submerging your body into water that's approximately 55 degrees can heal inflammation and help energize you. You can sample this method by taking a cold shower. Set the temp for as cool as you can stand in for 60 seconds.
3. **Essential oils.** Diffuse oils. Experiment with different oils to see what you like. Lavender helps with relaxation. Peppermint and eucalyptus open your sinuses.
4. **Resist the urge to work out.** When you're accustomed to some sort of physical exercise every day, it's hard to take even one day off. Depending on the course of the illness, recovery may dictate not working out for a week. Listen to your body. When you're tired, just rest. When I was really ill, I would take the laundry out of the washer, put it in the dryer, and lie down.
5. **Evaluate your life.** Is God telling you to slow down? This is a good opportunity to look at how effectively you spend your time. Chronic stress weakens the immune system.

MOVE FORWARD

Do the practice above that helped Ted rest despite the pain of double knee replacement surgery. Repeat this exercise throughout your day today. How did you feel after breathing the negativity or pain away?

PRAYER

Father God, I surrender my life to you. Use me. Wrap your arms around me and heal me. In Jesus's name I bind and cast out the spirit of infirmity. I rebuke it, Father! You are my mighty rock. My fortress. You have given me a strong and capable body—one that will do great things. I stand firm in your power and authority, knowing that in Jesus's name, true healing and restoration are mine. Amen.

DAY 20
WHEN NOTHING WORKS

"And let us not grow weary of doing good, for in due season we will reap, if we do not give up." Galatians 6:9

When you've tried every diet and nothing works, know you are not alone. The Centers for Disease Control and Prevention estimates that nearly half of adults in the United States tried to lose weight within the past year.*

Stepping onto the scale and seeing no reduction but possibly an increase is frustrating. Especially as we are certain we've done everything recommended. Spark healthy changes in your body with these three things: Increase the intensity, the frequency, and the duration with which you work out.

Intensity: Exercise harder, with short bursts of energetic movements. Try a H.I.I.T. workout. Engage your muscles, don't just go through the motions. Squat lower, deeper, and with intention.

Frequency: If you typically work out three days a week, work out four or five. Or commit to doing a few sit-ups and push-ups in the early mornings or evenings in addition to your regular workouts.

Duration: If you regularly exercise for thirty minutes, try forty-five, or even sixty.

Daily exercise is key. Find the thing that makes your heart sing and you'll do it more often. Walk, run, swim, dance—the type of movement does not matter. Moving matters. Mix up the variety. Just be sure to move every day for at least 15 minutes, preferably 30 or even 60.

Make sure you incorporate an even dose of cardio, toning, and stretching. When everything you're doing proves to be ineffective, make fitness a priority in your life.

---

* "Products—Data Briefs—Number 313—July 2018," Centers for Disease Control and Prevention, July 12, 2018, https://www.cdc.gov/nchs/products/databriefs/db313.htm#:~:text=Nearly%20one%2Dhalf%20(49.1%25),40–59%20(52.4%25).

Next, no one will lose weight and keep it off while continuing to eat unhealthy food. Say no to fast food, chemicals, and preservatives. I have found success in maintaining my weight with a carnivore diet that includes mostly protein like beef, venison, chicken, and fish; healthy fats like avocados and nuts; organic green vegetables like broccoli and asparagus, and occasionally fruit. Whatever diet works best for you, choose less-processed foods. The closer you get to the hoof, the soil, or the tree, the better the nutrition. Processed foods and foods cooked at high temperatures are nutrient-deficient. Because food is fuel for your body, fuel your body with superior fuel.

Do whatever you can to find the activities that make your heart sing and fill your day with those experiences as much as you can. If you want to get in shape, lose weight, and feel great but find yourself stuck, start with the basics like good old-fashioned exercise and a healthy diet. This might be all you need to start losing weight.

PERSEVERE

Despite results that are nonexistent or slow in coming, persevere with determination. Do the next right thing. Go to the gym. Avoid sugary snacks, sodas, chips, and fried food. Don't give up.

PEEL OFF POUNDS

Base every meal around protein and vegetables. Even breakfast. The average fruity smoothie contains about five teaspoons of sugar. Yes, I know, naturally-occurring sugar from fruit is healthier than refined sugars, but starting the day with mostly sugar in any form can send you crashing into fatigue within an hour.

Juice your morning beverage instead of blending. My favorite is made with spinach, beets, carrots, kale, ginger, and a green apple, which naturally contains less sugar than red apples.

If you're serious about losing weight, eliminate soda, candy, and cake, white flour, and white sugar. Limit alcohol consumption. Have a glass of wine or beer or cocktail but rather than having that second drink right away, have a big glass of water. Add slices of cucumber or lemon to your water.

Drink lots of water. You can set a reminder on your phone to notify you periodically throughout the day to drink water whether you need it or not. Sometimes we get busy and forget. Put lime or mint leaves in your water for a refreshing twist. You can also add fruit like strawberries, apples, or watermelon.

Get good sleep. Never miss an opportunity to rest. Sit outside on the rocking chair with your lemon water and just *be*.

Be careful of mindless eating and snacking. If you really want a piece of cake at a party, allow yourself to have a couple of bites. And don't fill up on the potato chips. Make good choices. All those excess unhealthy snacks will catch up, drag you down, and make you feel lethargic. When you go to a party, scan the room for healthy snacks and stay by those.

WORK OUT MORE EFFECTIVELY

If you're used to working out three days a week, taking the same Zumba or Spinning class, running or swimming, throw a brand-new workout into the mix. Your body will eventually adapt to the stress placed upon it as a means of survival if you choose the same activity, the same way week after week. By increasing the intensity, duration, or frequency of the workout, you confuse the muscles and make them stronger. More muscle means more calories burned at rest. Plus, you may discover a new exercise you like to do. After teaching group fitness classes for more than thirty years, I realize that by adding kickboxing and yoga into my weekly or monthly fitness routines, my body is more flexible and stronger.

BE HAPPIER

You can't just say you're going to be happier without having a plan. We all have stress. The challenge is to minimize the stress. Add activities that bring you joy and help others, too. Volunteer once a month at a children's hospital or animal shelter. During those precious moments, you won't be thinking about what you're having for dinner.

Add mindfulness and a mantra to your day. Set your phone alarm to alert you at random times throughout the day to breathe deeply and remind yourself of something positive. When the mindful alarm rings, slow whatever you're doing. If you're eating, chew more slowly. If you're sitting at your desk, close your eyes and take a deep breath. Do a mental body scan. In which areas do you hold more tension? Breathe.

At the beginning of each week, set random affirmation reminders about those things in life you appreciate like family, health, a job, a car, the sunshine. Big or small, what brings you joy?

MOVE FORWARD

As you reboot your commitment to improved health, don't be too hard on yourself if you miss a few days or a week. Tomorrow is another day. Begin again at the next opportunity.

PRAYER

God, you have given me this precious gift of a body. Help me to use it to its fullest potential so that I can be of service to others. I decree and declare this body is healthy and strong. You have given me authority to walk on snakes and scorpions. In Jesus's name I cut the cord to all ancestral curses in my life, now! Because of you, my body radiates perfect peace and confidence. In Jesus's mighty name, amen.

DAY 21
CULTIVATE CONFIDENCE

"Strength and dignity are her clothing, and she laughs at the time to come." Proverbs 31:25

When I was seven years old, my parents enrolled me in a YMCA swim team. When it was time for the beginners to learn the critical elements of competitive swimming, Coach Jack Lucas explained what we could expect. Swimming, I learned, was only half the battle. How we reacted to the bang of the starter's pistol was as important as kicking hard and using our arms to push and pull our bodies through the water.

Coach Jack yelled "bang" and we dove in, got out of the pool, and did it again. And a hundred times more.

PERSISTENCE

A study in the *Journal of Personality and Social Psychology* suggests that self-confidence is linked to better health, job performance, and overall well-being.[*] Interestingly, better health, job performance, and overall well-being is a confidence booster. Confidence is the result of knowing we have done something in the past and trust ourselves to do it again. It is also having faith.

What enables us to obtain a modicum of success at any endeavor is persistence. Do you give up the first time you try a new activity? In competitive swimming, there's a quiet moment when a referee instructs the participants to step onto the starting block. The crowd grows quiet as participants adjust their bathing suits, caps, and goggles.

Standing on the side of the pool is a referee with a starter pistol pointed in the air.

"Swimmers . . ." the referee yells. "Take your mark."

Swimmers bend and grab the edge of their starting block. Heads down, knees bent, muscles taut, they listen intently for the next command.

---

[*] Samantha Krauss and Ulrich Orth, "Work Experiences and Self-Esteem Development: A Meta-Analysis of Longitudinal Studies," *Sage Journals*, July 21, 2021, https://journals.sagepub.com/doi/full/10.1177/08902070211027142.

Bang! The pistol belches a thunderous crack, and swimmers catapult into the pool.

Having the courage to lurch into the cold water or into a new adventure is more than half the battle. The beginning of any activity is the first step toward gaining confidence and winning the raging war within.

If you commit to getting on the starting block of improved health, the planning and preparation pay off. Whether skiing, swimming, running, painting, singing, getting a degree, starting a new business, participating in a race, or cleaning out a closet, the most difficult task often is getting started.

Focusing on the past prevents you from living to your potential. Success and failure are based on trials and errors. Confidence comes from preparation, planning, persistence, and pausing a negative mindset.

If we never get up on that starting block and at least try something, we may never know the joy God has in store. *Reframe* your approach to whatever battle you're fighting and you'll likely see a new outcome. What if we were to apply the same *Bang!* technique as mentioned from the swimming story to a new exercise program? What if we looked at failure in a positive light? After all, someone who fails is in process. What if you gave yourself enough grace to argue that you can be successful despite age, energy level, or other responsibilities?

Research shows that our brains have the capacity for learning and growth throughout our lives. During adolescence, we learn new behavior, language, and emotions almost daily. The neural pathways in our brains are soft and pliable like warm taffy. The more we engage in physical and intellectual experiences, the more the neurons in our brains create connections or synapses. As the years go by, we do activities with which we are comfortable and familiar, and so our rate of learning diminishes, as does our confidence.

Bestselling author and neurologist Dr. David Perlmutter states, "The ability of the brain to change and reorganize itself and its function is called neuroplasticity. Neuroplasticity provides us with a brain that can adapt not only to changes inflicted by damage, but more importantly, allows adaptation to any and all experiences and changes we may encounter."[*]

EMBRACE YOUR IDENTITY

Starting a new job or hobby stimulates brain activity and gives a sense of accomplishment and confidence.

Gain courage and confidence with small, concise steps. Inquire about lessons for whatever activity you'd like to try. Search the internet for groups or instructors in your area to learn how to ride a horse, paint, sing, play an instrument, get in shape, or plant a garden. There are highly qualified people who would love to share their gifts and talents. You just have to ask.

---

[*]   David Perlmutter, "The Process of Neuroplasticity and Making New Connections," *David Perlmutter M.D.,* September 23, 2013, https://www.drperlmutter.com/process-neuroplasticity/.

Discovering an exciting new hobby that ignites your spirit opens your senses to personal growth, happiness, and confidence. Experiences can also show us what we don't want in our lives. Deconstructing dreams leads to becoming more authentic and confident. Having traveled to Africa, I recall what it feels like to see a herd of zebra in their natural habitat, the coral-colored dirt, the unbearably hot sun, and the amazing smiles of our host Dr. Rocco Gioia and the workers on his fifty-thousand-acre tomato ranch in Hoedspruit. At night, we'd sit outside at a lapa—an open-air fire pit—sipping African wine by the crackling fire, listening to hippos and hyena making noises nearby. Those memories buoy my spirit.

Synapses in our brain are at work making connections when we recall memories. The more we think and learn and physically move our bodies, the greater chance we have for improving memory, focus, and our health. On one of our trips to Africa when my son was a toddler, Dr. Rocco Gioia and I watched young Rocco play with building blocks, infatuated with the angles and colors of the blocks.

"He's not just playing," Dr. Rocco observed. "He's working."

Confidence comes partially from experiences teaching what has worked in the past, and how we felt in certain situations, environments, and in the presence of others. We receive the blessing of courage and confidence through the gifts of the Holy Spirit: wisdom, understanding, counsel, fortitude, knowledge, piety, and fear of the Lord. We gain assurance and understanding to make decisions through His grace.

Our confidence is elevated when we have healthy relationships with family, friends, and coworkers. Conversely, one snarky comment can feel like a gut punch from Mike Tyson. Some relationships can be effortless and uplifting, while interactions with others are irritating. Family members raised in the same household become two different people with opposing viewpoints. We develop self-preservation tools to combat bullies, to be loved, or to get attention.

Unknowingly, children learn survival mechanisms. Pouting or withholding affection may have helped us get what we needed, but carrying those behaviors into adult years masks who we are at our core. Constantly trying to please others is exhausting. Trust me. We cover wounds in our souls with happy faces while screaming inside. We camouflage thoughts to appear to be in control. At times, we portray an image of what we think others expect while sacrificing our souls. Then we wonder why we lack confidence.

God has given gifts and talents. Some people are more introverted and prefer working alone. Others are more outgoing and love to take center stage. Neither is better or worse. Introverts need extroverts and vice versa. An actor might be good at performing on stage and rely on someone to help with taxes. The person crunching numbers all day needs to forget about balance sheets and go to a play. We need one another.

MOVE FORWARD

I never realized how unhappy I was until I nearly died from toxic mold exposure. It isn't easy, but how can you *reframe* current and past predicaments? What activities, or even clothes, make you feel confident?

PRAYER

Dear Lord, when situations beyond our control become so overwhelming that we lose hope, guide us back to finding confidence in you. Remind me today that you are always near, always my strength. As you tell us in Isaiah 41:10, "Fear not, for I am with you; be not dismayed, for I am your God; I will strengthen you, I will help you, I will uphold you with my righteous right hand." My deepest desire is to serve you with wild confidence. In Jesus's name, amen.

DAY 22
SWEAT & SWEAT EQUITY

"His master said to him, 'Well done, good and faithful servant. You have been faithful over a little; I will set you over much. Enter into the joy of your master.'" Matthew 25:23

By eight o'clock that night the temperature had dropped slightly but was still a sweltering one hundred and five degrees. My husband, Ted, was about to get on stage and perform a ninety-minute, fiercely energetic concert outdoors. The fact that he was seventy-four years old worried me a bit.

"Here," I pushed a can into his hands. "Be sure to hydrate with extra water and this post-workout drink. You'll need the electrolytes and minerals."

Sadly, he forgot to take the drink on stage with him.

While the fingers of his left hand danced wildly on the neck of the guitar, his right hand grasped a pick, rapidly strumming chords. I watched from the side of the stage as a pool of sweat grew at his feet. With his arms dripping from perspiration, his hands and fingers saturated and slippery, I wondered how it was possible for him to hold his pick and hit every single note flawlessly. To emphasize key crescendos in a song, he'd lunge low, even after having two knee replacements.

"He's done all this a million times before," I told myself. Tonight, he had skin in the game. Sweat equity.

Having performed more than six thousand concerts over sixty years, Ted was used to playing in the heat, the cold, in large stadiums, and small theaters. Nothing phased him. He spent decades rehearsing, practicing, playing, and doing the exhaustive but rewarding work of mastering his musical craft. He had conquered any and all physical and environmental terrain.

The difference between Ted's guitar playing and someone who is starting to play are two things: sweat and sweat equity. Matthew 7:16 says, "You will recognize them by their fruits." Ted has invested an extensive portion of his life practicing and mastering his craft, and it shows.

Similarly, actor Mark Wahlberg is in phenomenal shape with an eight-pack of abs he shows constantly on social media. Mark works out daily and sticks to a strict diet. While there are other interpretations of this Bible verse, we can apply the words to recognize the result of how hard both men have worked at their crafts. They are dedicated and have relentless commitment.

We can all single out individuals who are serious about staying in shape. No matter how busy they are with work and family, they carve out time to spend at the gym. They eliminate junk food that sabotages their goals. Are you willing to make that commitment?

Despite our best intentions, some of us are not willing to choose a lifestyle that fosters good health. We have other priorities. Ecclesiastes 3:1 reminds, "For everything there is a season, and a time for every matter under heaven." When our children are young, extra workouts are not our first concern. When they grow up and move on and out, we have a few extra hours per week to fit in a Zumba or Pilates class. Only two things separate us from looking like the toned people parading around the gym: sweat and sweat equity. We have to make time.

If I had to pinpoint one thing that helped me stay in shape and combat the signs of aging, it's breaking a sweat during a workout. In the winter I heat my workout room with a portable infrared heater to eighty-five degrees. Like Ted has played concerts in extreme temperatures and tolerates it, I've enjoyed dancing, stretching, and toning exercises in warmer rooms for decades. My muscles are more limber and easier to stretch, I burn more calories, and feel as though I'm more exhausted and satiated. Heated workouts are not for everyone. Gradually work your way up to warmer temperatures and see if you can tolerate and enjoy the experience. Some people cannot sweat because of toxic build-up or beta blockers. If heated workouts aren't resonating with you, it may be beneficial for you to take a cold plunge first, then go into a steam or infrared sauna. Go back and forth several times.

Detoxifying the body through sweat removes impurities and improves complexion, circulation, and mental focus. Be sure, however, to hydrate adequately. Too much of a good thing, in this case, isn't always good.

The time, energy, and effort you put into strength training, cardiovascular exercise, and stretching will ultimately bring big results. Flex your muscles in the gym, do the splits at seventy, or dance like no one is watching.

MOVE FORWARD

Try exercising until you get a good sweat going.

PRAYER

God, I humbly ask for you to help me make healthy living and eating a priority in my life. I love you, worship you, and desire to make you Lord of my life. I falter and I cave into the deception that I am too busy to exercise and sweat. All I want is to hear, "Well done, good and faithful servant." Guide my steps, Father. In Jesus's name I pray, amen.

DAY 23
SPIRITUAL WARFARE

"For we do not wrestle against flesh and blood, but against the rulers, against the authorities, against the cosmic powers over this present darkness, against the spiritual forces of evil in the heavenly places." Ephesians 6:12

Not until I was in my fifties did I start to understand and recognize spiritual warfare. When I was writing a book titled *Killer House*, I was fascinated to rediscover the verses in Leviticus that pertained to mold. A creative non-fiction, *Killer House* details my life-threatening illness from toxic mold growing between the walls of my MTV Cribs home.

We demolished the house and moved to Texas. Then, we had a water leak in our home. We built a new home and, although we emphasized the need to construct a state-of-the-art structure that wouldn't leak, there were four water leaks before we moved in. Insurance didn't cover the cost of our repairs.

Why was water following me, making me and my family sick, and creating financial destruction? In Jennifer LeClaire's book, *Defeating Water Spirits*, I found answers. "Demons," LeClaire writes, "try to choke you—or put you in a stranglehold."

Could a demonic force be trying to snare, defeat, and sicken us? Jennifer goes on, "Translating this to our spiritual realities, the enemy wants to choke the Word of God out of your mouth so you can't wield your sword of the Spirit or pray." I wanted to learn more.

WHAT IS SPIRITUAL WARFARE?

Spiritual warfare is a physical symptom of a spiritual battle. Right now, there is an invisible war waging between good and evil—between God and his enemy, Satan. What some may not realize, is that the war is at your door, in your home and community, everywhere, twenty-four hours a day. Any way that Satan can steal your joy, cause chaos, and tempt you, he will. Satan lays in wait for the right moment to plunge us into doubting our faith and to steal us away from God. This unseen spiritual war affects you, your family, friends, and everyone you encounter every moment. "For he will deliver you from the snare of the fowler and from the deadly pestilence," Psalm 91:3.

Satan's army is ready to entrap through any means necessary, especially through our weaknesses and addictions. Cupcakes and cookies seem like an unlikely place, but consider how you feel after devouring a whole pizza instead of one slice. Five cookies instead of one?

A whole bag of chips rather than a handful? The Bible warns about overindulging and being gluttons in Proverbs 28:7: "The one who keeps the law is a son with understanding, but a companion of gluttons shames his father." When the pursuit and pleasure of eating becomes our focus, we have given into the temptation and missed the mark.

As an archer, I've spent hundreds, if not thousands, of hours shooting my bow, aiming for the bull's-eye in the target. Even with years of practice I usually miss the mark, even if just by a millimeter. The word *sin* comes from the Greek word *hamartia*, which means to miss the mark. Every day we miss the mark in parenting, relationships, work, and taking care of our health. We get busy and fail to make exercise a priority. We trade healthy, whole foods for prepackaged snacks with empty calories. We overeat at Thanksgiving and on the weekends because that little voice in the back of our mind says, "You've worked hard. You deserve it."

You may not struggle with what you think of as addictions or temptations—pornography, drugs, or alcohol—but what about overeating? Have you considered that Satan has ensnared you through food?

Over the years I've attended dozens of different churches. Most pastors do not preach about spiritual warfare and weapons to fight the devil. "Milquetoast Christianity" refers to believers who are lukewarm and rarely engage in deep discussions about religion, politics, or spirituality. God instructs us to put on the armor and be battle-ready. We have been given tools to fight the devil's fiery darts with warfare, shields of protection, God's word, and prayer. "He, however, shook off the creature into the fire and suffered no harm," Acts 28:5.

Spiritual attacks come in many forms, from illness to loss of income, even water infiltration that destroys your home. The devil entices lukewarm Christians to break down, give up, and cross over to the enemy camp. Frankly, he is doing a decent job. How many in your own circle of family and friends are unbelievers? In mine, there are still many.

We know, however, in the end, God wins. Until then, we put on the armor of God and shield ourselves. Find a pastor who will train and equip you with knowledge of warfare. Be bold and brave. Have faith.

"For we do not wrestle against flesh and blood, but against the rulers, against the authorities, against the cosmic powers over this present darkness, against the spiritual forces of evil in the heavenly places. Therefore take up the whole armor of God, that you may be able to withstand in the evil day, and having done all, to stand firm. Stand therefore, having fastened on the belt of truth, and having put on the breastplate of righteousness, and, as shoes for your feet, having put on the readiness given by the gospel of peace. In all circumstances take up the shield of faith, with which you can extinguish all the flaming darts of the evil one; and take the helmet of salvation, and the sword of the Spirit, which is the word of God," Ephesians 6:13–17.

Satan can attack your:

- Confidence
- Emotions

- Energy
- Health
- Finances
- Fitness
- Joy
- Relationships
- Weight loss

His tools include:

- Ancestral curses
- Casting spells
- Magic
- Mediums and psychics
- Palm reading
- Pharmaceutical drugs (aka: sorcery[*])
- Pornography
- Sorcery
- Toxic environments and relationships
- Unhealthy habits
- Witchcraft
- Worshiping other gods

Yet, God has not left us defenseless. He has equipped us with weapons of warfare:

- Casting out demons
- Decrees and declarations
- Deliverance
- Fasting
- Praise and worship music
- Prayer
- Prayer plus fasting
- Prayer plus healing touch
- Reading scripture

---

[*] "G5331—Pharmakeia—Strong's Greek Lexicon (KJV)," Blue Letter Bible, accessed October 25, 2023, https://www.blueletterbible.org/lexicon/g5331/kjv/tr/0-1/.

MOVE FORWARD

Begin to notice how spiritual warfare is operating in your life. Just as you would search for a medical doctor to help with a minor illness or the best surgeon to perform a life-saving surgery, search for an experienced pastor to advise you about your next steps. Perhaps deliverance is needed, but whoever you choose for guidance will basically be performing spiritual surgery on you. Proceed with caution. Do your homework. The situation could be made worse by well-meaning people who aren't properly equipped to do this important work. Check the Resources (page 161) for recommended spiritual warfare training and books.

PRAYER

God, I thank you for this reminder that with you all things are possible. You have given me authority to cast out demons, and today, I decree and declare in the name of Jesus, no unclean spirit enters my life, my family's lives, or my community. I bind them in the name of Jesus and cast them into the lake of fire! I break the ties of ancestral curses in my life. Satan isn't welcome in my home! I place a bloodline of protection around this room, my home, my property, and my family. Wrap your arms around me. Protect me from the evil one. Send your warring angels in front of me and guide my steps. In Jesus's mighty name, amen.

DAY 24
SKIN CARE

"Charm is deceptive, and beauty is fleeting, but a woman who fears the Lord is to be praised."
Proverbs 31:30

I wanted to call off the whole thing. There was no way I could be seen in public. Maybe I could postpone the event. But people were flying in for the day and wanted to celebrate *with me*. But not when I looked like you could play connect the dots on my face. Running my fingertips gently down my cheeks, I felt the little bumps everywhere.

Why now and what is this anyway? Chicken pox? Shingles? A dozen or more tiny red pimple-like dots covered my face one week before my sixtieth birthday party. There's only one chance to be sixty. No do-overs.

As a teenager, I didn't really have acne. A few breakouts here and there, but nothing outrageous. After the birth of my son, in my late twenties, I started getting cystic acne. My dermatologist said they were probably from hormonal fluctuations. Those shockingly huge bumps were difficult to conceal and there were times when I did stay home until they went away with topical treatments or injections.

At least these bumps were smaller and I could cover them with makeup. I had to make a decision: Do I cancel my sixtieth birthday party because of the way I look?

As we age, we encounter a variety of skin issues mostly due to hormonal changes, allergic reactions, and what we eat. We grab the first, highest-rated anti-aging products we find, or those recommended by our doctor, or a friend. But we're not just dealing with wrinkles and fine lines. Natural aging also includes hyperpigmentation, saggy skin, dryness, age spots, enlarged pores, skin tags, cancer, and what I discovered I had just before my birthday: rosacea.

Stress can wreak havoc on your body. Throwing sparks to the kindling are a lack of sleep, poor eating and exercise habits, and even the air we breathe. There are environmental factors that cause skin rashes, such as exposure to toxic mold, pollution, and—how can we forget—poison ivy. Genetics plays a big role too.

My dermatologist put me on topical ointment and an antibiotic specifically for rosacea. I also took a steroid dose pack, and my skin cleared enough for me to enjoy the party. I battled with rosacea for the next few months, then found switching my face cream helped immensely.

There isn't one way to fix all our skin care issues, especially with skin that is designed by God to show the outward expression of a life lived well. Crow's feet and deep crevices around our mouth and between our eyebrows show we've experienced sorrow, love, and joy. While I have had botox to soften wrinkles, it is often overdone or improperly done. Botox is poison. It freezes your muscles so they can't move. Side effects can be droopy lids, bruising, headaches, flu-like symptoms, and infection.

Whether to get plastic surgery, a face lift, or injections to lift cheeks or plump lips is a personal decision. Every day I wake up, look in the mirror, and at times I'm okay with the brown spots and less-taut skin on my face. Other days, it bothers me more.

Then I see a beautiful, gray-haired woman with an engaging smile that exudes confidence, and I suddenly love her wrinkles. She possesses a subtle elegance and obvious charm. There is an inviting grace and wisdom etched on her face. Why would anyone want to take that away? "Wisdom is with the aged, and understanding in length of days," Job 12:12.

BEAUTY FROM WITHIN

The best skin care starts from within and is instantly recognizable. When you feel that inner joy that only a relationship with God can provide, it shows on your skin. Aging gracefully is accepting the changes in our bodies with a positive attitude. That doesn't mean we can't slow the process and take care to hide a few imperfections.

Flawless, poreless, unblemished skin is almost unattainable as we approach our golden years. Years of stress and sun worship become visible, but more often to us than others. Combatting the spots and wrinkles takes diligence and time. Finding a good esthetician and getting facials regularly are key, but who has time? And that's the problem, isn't it? When we're too busy, too stressed, and neglect our health, the results show on our faces.

Wherever you are, you can find results when you give attention to your skin. Begin with taking care of what's going on beneath your skin.

- Make prayer and gratitude an integral part of your life.
- Heal your body from the inside out. Exercise daily and get a good sweat going in your workout at least twice a week to flush out the impurities in your skin.
- Eliminate fried foods, fast food, white flour, and sugar.
- Drink more water.

It's nearly impossible to eliminate toxic chemicals from the cosmetics and lotions we slather on our faces and bodies. Careful research will find products that are made from natural ingredients. Going *au natural* with coconut and rose oil is an option. Pure coconut oil and pure almond oil can be applied directly to moisten and nourish skin from head to toe. Use enough to rub into skin but not so much to feel oily. The products I use that solve my skin issues might not accomplish your goals, so experiment and listen to your body to know what is best for your skin. The various settings and seasons of life may require adjustments to your routine.

My skin care routine begins with drinking a glass of water as soon as I wake up. After sleeping through the night, our body is dehydrated, so that first glass carries necessary hydration through our system and helps with detoxification.

Next, I splash my face with cold water and dab a bit of Shiseido eye cream under my eyes, followed by Celletoi Youth Serum all over my face. I let out the dogs to do their own morning routine and make coffee. Several times a week, while I go through my morning chores, I put on a detoxifying, organic mud mask. After I tend to emails, take care of business, and vacuum dog hair, I get creative and spend an hour or two writing. With a portable infrared heater, an hour before I plan to exercise, I start warming up my workout room so when it's time to move, I break a sweat. Sweating, I believe, is a critical element to skin wellness.

After a shower, I use Celletoi cleanser and wipe an Elemis peel pad on my face to remove dead skin cells and lessen brown spots. Then I follow up with eye cream, serum, and Celletoi face cream. To relieve puffiness and massage my face, I use a jade roller. Now my face is ready for a little makeup—or not. When I can, I allow the skin on my face to breathe *sans* makeup. While I go through phases, at the moment I have eyelash extensions, which cuts my prep time in half. Next, a little concealer under my eyes and on brown spots, then a light touch of organic foundation powder, bronzer, fill in brows, lip gloss, and I'm done.

MOVE FORWARD

If you don't have access to a sauna, make a date to visit a spa that offers organic facials and has a sauna you can relax in before or after the treatment. From the bulleted list, what one item will you begin today? Which can you apply next?

PRAYER

Father God, I come to you today so humbled and grateful. There are moments when I become too self-conscious, forgetting to embrace and love the skin I'm in. These insecurities sometimes cloud my vision, taking my focus away from you. Lord, free me from these distractions and let my eyes remain steadfastly on you. May I find comfort and acceptance in the way in which I'm beautifully and wonderfully made in your image. Help me to embrace my skin and not be ashamed of tiny flaws. Help me to see myself—gray hair, wrinkly skin, and all—as you see me. Sometimes I get so wrapped up in my own insecurities that I lose focus. Release me from anything that takes my eyes off you. In Jesus's name, amen.

DAY 25
FINDING PURPOSE

"Love your neighbor as yourself." Matthew 22:39

We appreciate our health most when we're sidelined with sniffles or an illness much worse. Simple things like folding laundry become monumental tasks. When I lost my health so dramatically, I realized how fortunate I was to recover. Daily, I appreciate having enough energy to not only climb stairs, but to work out, love my family, and teach others how to have a healthier and happier life. I take extra precautions to avoid the foods and behaviors that make me feel less than amazing, and I've become more adventurous.

As our kids get older and less dependent on us, it's time to put our own needs first whenever possible. If you're in a good mood, others might be more inclined to follow your lead. Fill your happy cup all the way. Rediscover those things that you enjoyed as a child in a way that's safe and healthy.

Perhaps you loved to jump on the trampoline and every time you drive by one of those trampoline facilities geared toward school-age kids, you imagine how it would feel to be silly and jump on the trampoline again. When you remind yourself of your age, however, the idea of giving it a try quickly fades.

The American Psychological Association found that having a sense of purpose in life is associated with a lower risk of mortality and cardiovascular diseases. In my experience, purpose is connected to living life in a fashion that helps others.

Boston University School of Public Health (BUSPH) researchers found that people with higher levels of purpose may have a lower risk of death from any cause.[*] Possessing a high sense of purpose in life is associated with a reduced risk for all-cause mortality and cardiovascular events. According to a survey by Pew Research Center, 26 percent of US adults say they think about the meaning and purpose of life on a daily basis. What makes life meaningful? Where do Americans find meaning in life?

The importance of finding purpose in our lives is strongly linked to helping others. In Matthew 22:37–39, Jesus outlined the two greatest commandments: "'Love the Lord your God with all your heart and with all your soul and with all your mind.' This is the first and greatest commandment. And the second is like it: 'Love your neighbor as yourself.'"

---

[*] "Higher Sense of Purpose in Life May Be Linked to Lower Mortality Risk, Study Finds," ScienceDaily, November 15, 2022, https://www.sciencedaily.com/releases/2022/11/221115184500.htm.

Additionally, there is a strong association between life purpose and mortality among US adults older than fifty years.[*] Unleashing supernatural health means exploring health as a catalyst for Divine Purpose. The resulting abundant energy is channeled to pursue passions, share God's word, and employ gifts and talents to assist others.

When we live authentically rooted in a desire to be happy, fulfilled, and valuable to God, our family, friends, and others, that happiness seeps into every aspect of our lives. Interactions with strangers at the grocery store become kinder and more thoughtful. We smile more. Something seemingly so small like a friendly gesture can create a huge ripple effect for changing the lives of others. When you live your life in a way that makes you joyful and purposeful, you are a catalyst for change.

Finding purpose can be challenging for some, especially those who've been living their lives to please others.

Diet, exercise, prayer, and meditation are important elements in maintaining a positive attitude even when everything seems to be going wrong and everyone seems to be out to get us. First, the food we ingest can give us energy or zap it. The way we move and stretch our bodies contributes to physical wellness. By following our bliss, we can *reawaken* a joyful, childlike attitude. Having a greater awareness for and connection with God restores our faith. And faith gives us hope that God is with us on this journey.

When you aren't fulfilling your God-given destiny, however, it may feel like you're missing out on something.

Of course, learning about personalities helped me to better understand more about myself and why I feel at ease with some people and why others push my buttons. It's interesting to see how two people react differently to the same situation. It has opened my eyes so intensely that when someone disagrees with me or treats me in a way that is vastly different than I would prefer, instead of instinctively reacting with anger, I softly smile. I get it. Each of us is doing the best we can with the information and childhood wounds we've experienced.

MOVE FORWARD

Make a list of skills that come easily for you and that bring you joy. Next, find a charity in your area that could benefit from your gifts and talents.

PRAYER

Father, I praise you for the many gifts, talents, and skills with which I've been blessed. Help me to use them for your kingdom purposes. In Jesus's name, amen.

---

[*]   Aliya Alimujiang, Ashley Wiensch, and Jonathan Boss, "Association between Life Purpose and Mortality among US Adults Older than 50 Years," JAMA Network Open, May 24, 2019, https://jamanetwork .com/journals/jamanetworkopen/fullarticle/2734064.

DAY 26
GROW YOUR OWN

"... I will restore the fortunes of my people Israel,
and they shall rebuild the ruined cities and inhabit them;
they shall plant vineyards and drink their wine,
and they shall make gardens and eat their fruit."
Amos 9:14

I never understood what the hype was about until I experienced gardening for myself. Truthfully, I didn't have a green thumb. It's one thing to grow herbs in small pots on the kitchen windowsill or have a couple of potted plants in the living room that need water twice a week. But to build a garden, cultivate the soil, and plant the seeds was downright daunting.

For a few years I started small and grew tomatoes, basil, rosemary, kale, and squash in a portable and easy to use Vegepod I saw advertised online. Picking out the location, I discovered, is a critical element to successfully grow a garden.

1. Location. Initially, I positioned the portable raised garden stand conveniently outside my back door. In the Texas summer heat, however, that particular corner turned out to be a sauna and not conducive to nurturing plants. Fortunately, the portable planter was easily movable to another location that had afternoon sun and breeze. The resulting tomatoes, kale, and basil burst with flavor.
2. Get help. Having the guidance and expertise of an experienced gardener is helpful. Our ranch hand, Bobby, and his wife, Sara, successfully gardened for years, so along with Rocco and his girlfriend, Bell, we built four raised beds four feet wide and eight feet long. While Bobby did most of the heavy work excavating a thirty-two-square-foot area on our property (I did run the tractor once), we put up an eight-foot fence so deer and other wildlife could not raid the plants. Sara researched the nutrients essential for soil in our geographic location and we discussed what vegetables and herbs we wanted.
3. Reap what you sow. "For whatever one sows, that will he also reap," says Galatians 6:7.

The seeds sprouted within days! Walking in the garden each morning, I was amazed at what had grown overnight. Squash blossoms opened in the early morning hours as the sun shined through the leaves. The subtle progression of vegetables peeking through the soil made me smile. With God's help, we produced food that would nourish our family! Tiny squash vines expanded and reached higher weekly, so we put up trellises that connected one garden bed to another. The tomato, watermelon, and squash vines exploded, climbing up the archway within a week.

"You have to see my garden," I told those who visited as if I had just gotten a new puppy. I encouraged them to pick a sweet baby tomato along with a pungent basil leaf, like a mini caprese salad. I'd clip lavender, rosemary, squash, peppers, and kale for guests to take home.

Along with the sense of accomplishment and satisfaction that comes from growing your own vegetables, spending time outdoors and getting your hands in the dirt relieves stress and anxiety. Nothing is more peaceful than being surrounded by nature and enveloped by God's great many wonders. Trees gently dancing in the breeze, a million different hues of green, and the backdrop of a bright blue sky can be instantly calming. It's also a wonderful place to talk to God.

Growing your own herbs and vegetables is not only healthy, but gardening can lower your blood pressure, increase your vitamin D level, improve your mood, and combat loneliness.

MOVE FORWARD

Start small and check out a portable garden planter where you can plant herbs, tomatoes, and easy to grow vegetables. The soil makes a difference and so does your geographic location and time of year to plant. There are many resources available online for gardening in your area.

PRAYER

Heavenly Father, thank you for the blessing of fragrant herbs and nutritious vegetables. I am grateful for the sunshine, the rain, and the combination of elements that make me appreciate your perfect design. Let our garden be abundant. Grace me with the knowledge and wisdom to cultivate and grow my own vegetables. I love you, Father, and praise you. In Jesus's mighty name, amen.

DAY 27
LONGEVITY

"With long life I will satisfy him and show him my salvation." Psalm 91:16

"Are you ready?" I asked.

Rocco stood patiently on the trampoline next to me. "Ready, Mom."

In my mind, I was fifteen again, effortlessly going through the motions: Jump three times, reach arms overhead, then bring your knees up to your chest. I'd done a backflip on a trampoline hundreds of times throughout my adolescence, but could I still do this move at fifty-five?

I bounced slowly, gradually jumping with more strength and energy each time. "One, two, three," I yelled.

On the third bounce my arms flew over my head, I tucked my knees into my hands and flipped backwards in the air.

"Good job," Rocco acknowledged.

When I see healthy and fit senior citizens like Sister Madonna Buder who completed triathlons in her eighties, I feel as though I could be doing more. Even if we eat a well-balanced diet free of chemicals and preservatives and we don't drink or smoke, we're still in the running for a disease or medical condition that reduces life span. So how can we enhance the quality and vitality of our lives and live as long as possible?

GEOGRAPHY

Blue Zones identify regions around the globe where the life expectancy is longer than the average population. What do they eat and what is their lifestyle individually and as a community? Sardinia, Italy; Okinawa, Japan; Loma Linda, California; Nicoya Peninsula, Costa Rica; and Ikaria, Greece are a few Blue Zone cities.

Common denominators include they enjoy gardening, daily walks in sunshine, and regularly do low-impact exercise. Their lives are filled with a sense of purpose and belonging. They don't have busy lifestyles filled with appointments and deadlines. Here's the good news—they take naps and have happy hour.

While overall their stress is moderate, that's not to say they don't suffer loss or difficult times. Their faith, however, helps them endure. They enjoy the same approach to life, exercise, and food that I've encouraged on social media, in my online programs, and here in this book: the 80/20 Lifestyle. People in Blue Zones eat predominantly nutrient-dense foods and stop eating when they're mostly full. They prioritize faith and spending time with family and friends. They eat fresh vegetables and have a positive outlook on life. And yes, they occasionally indulge.

GENETICS

Genetics plays a role in our aging process, but minimally. You may have parents and grand-parents who live to become centenarians, but if you consume only white bread, hot dogs, sodas, and what is considered to be the average Western diet, you'll speed up the aging clock significantly. But not always.

Rolling Stones guitarist Keith Richards has lived a long rockstar life indulging in drinking, smoking, and recreational drugs as he described in his memoir, *Life*. Sometimes life is a mystery, randomly mixing up the answers to confuse us, or perhaps just to keep us guessing, striving, and working for solutions. Scientists have been scrambling to find cures for Alzheimer's disease, cancer, diabetes, and heart disease, many of which are linked to stress and poor diet choices.

COMMON INFLUENCERS FOR LONGEVITY

- Consume mostly nutrient-dense foods
- Cut out excess carbs, fast food, GMO's, sugar, soda, preservatives, and food dyes
- Move your body daily, especially if you have a sedentary job or lifestyle
- Avoid late night snacking
- Fast or minimize quantity of food
- Add strength training, cardio exercise, and stretching to your workouts
- Find creative outlets like painting, reading, writing, or gardening
- Make faith a significant part of your life
- Find an event or organization to volunteer your time
- Have a social life
- Minimize stress
- Get quality sleep
- Spend time with family
- Do something exciting or adventurous
- Have a pet
- Minimize cell phone and social media use
- Try an infrared sauna followed by a cold plunge or cold shower

- Stay hydrated
- Have a positive and grateful attitude
- Dance as if no one is watching

MOVE FORWARD

Which actions from the above list can you include in your schedule today? How can you embrace the positives in your life right now?

PRAYER

Father God, you have called me to do great things, and I know that you are always with me. You bear the weight of my burdens, and for that I'm so grateful. My blessings are abundant. I cherish each and every moment here and desire an eternity with you. Thank you for loving me. In Jesus's name, amen.

DAY 28
FUNCTIONAL MEDICINE

*"Heal me, O Lord, and I shall be healed; save me, and I shall be saved,
for you are my praise." Jeremiah 17:14*

Laying in a dark and quiet room, I breathed through an oxygen mask while vitamins dripped into my body through an IV. When my chest felt like an elephant sat there, I feared I was having a heart attack and Ted had rushed me to the hospital. Yet my chest x-rays and other tests were clear. Emergency Room doctors couldn't find a cause for my symptoms. The countless prescriptions I took caused other problems and did little to heal my body. Hope and healing came in the form of functional medicine, which strives to find the root cause of a disease.

After a toxicologist diagnosed me with having pre-emphysema and four different types of mold in my bloodstream, he recommended I go to Dallas and get treatment from Dr. William Rea at the Environmental Health Center. Dr. Rea wanted to get me off all medication and find out if there were foods or pollen that could be exacerbating some of my symptoms. He prescribed a rotation diet, suggesting I eat only one item, maybe two, at each meal such as chicken and broccoli, and then eliminate those items from my diet for four days. With this system, each particular food has a chance to be digested completely and I could track the slightest physical reaction to what I ate.

Of course, I gave up sugar, fried food, fast food, soda, alcohol, preservatives, and anything that wasn't fresh. Tracking my food intake and reactions, allergy testing, and supplements became my full-time job.

The detoxifying treatments at the Environmental Health Center produced my hoped-for results. For the first time in years, the fog that shrouded my brain lifted. I slept well, enjoyed more energy, and the constant migraines subsided.

Dr. Rea's functional medicine protocol was unconventional. The health and wellness industry generates 18 billion dollars yearly in the United States alone to cover pharmaceutical drugs that temporarily address symptoms. But masking symptoms does not heal an ailing body or eliminate the source of the illness and pain.

At the clinic, we discussed my symptoms including chronic fatigue, digestive problems, heart palpitations, insomnia, joint pain, restless legs, and skin rashes. The most debilitating were the migraines.

Seeking causes for these ailments, the doctor conducted allergy testing for everything from vinegar to cedar trees to camel meat since I had been to Africa several times.

While in residence, my daily protocol included fifteen to twenty minutes on an indoor bicycle. I'd down a mixture of psyllium and tri-salts, a large glass of filtered water, then spend twenty minutes in an infrared sauna. After a shower, I had a massage designed to drain my lymphatic system. Then I'd get an IV with vitamins and minerals while also receiving pure oxygen.

Although Dr. Rea recommended I continue the holistic treatments at the facility for three months, I missed my son. After nearly four weeks, I felt 50 percent better and ready to go home. Nurses taught me how to give myself immunotherapy injections of glutathione and histamine at home, but I was worried. Would being in the real world of toxins, chemical scents, and mold send me into a tailspin of brain fog, headaches, and fatigue? I had learned that residual effects of mold exposure could stay with me for months or years.

HOME AGAIN

Back home, I had to reacclimate to the toxins in the environment in and around my house. When we decided to move to Central Texas, we didn't consider the pollinating seasons. At the first sign of a winter cold front, a greenish yellow powder exploded from the cedar trees on our property causing a runny nose, sore throat, coughing, and headaches. Knowing how to give myself allergy shots proved critical to treat cedar fever.

I continued supplements and shots, juiced every day, purchased an infrared sauna, and ordered oxygen tanks to continue those treatments. I encouraged Ted to do oxygen treatments at home and while on tour. A friend who was a nurse administered vitamin IVs.

Always involved in Rocco's education and after-school activities, I felt eager to meet his new teachers. But coming into the school felt akin to being struck by a truck barreling at breakneck speed. Cleansing my body from toxins keenly awakened my sense of smell to the slightest noxious odor. Covering my nose with my shirtsleeve, I hustled into the front office, explained my unfortunate condition, and asked if the teachers could meet with me outside in the sunshine and fresh air.

A few times I slipped back into ill health after leaving the Environmental Health Center. Some family and friends understood my sensitivities. A few didn't, and I recognized the sneering looks when visitors saw Ted and I laying on the couch with oxygen masks.

Months later, I could go into a mall or restaurant without repercussions. Nearly twenty years later, I get vitamin IVs every few months containing magnesium, glutathione, vitamin C, zinc, and saline.

The Centers for Disease Control and Prevention states that nearly half of all adults in the United States have at least one chronic disease.[*] Exposure to toxic mold or other inflammatory illnesses triggers chemical sensitivity. Alternative remedies or functional medicine such as acupuncture, infrared sauna, massage for lymphatic drainage, oxygen therapy, vitamin IV, and eliminating chemicals from home and diet slowly detoxify the body and lead to feeling better. Natural healing isn't a quick fix. Sometimes improvement may take several months to notice any benefit.

MOVE FORWARD

When possible, see if holistic remedies can effectively partner with your body's natural healing abilities. Prescription drugs that mask the body's symptoms may be a temporary relief, but the root cause the symptoms are warning about are best addressed and fixed for lasting recovery and improved lifestyle. Search for a functional medicine doctor near you.

PRAYER

Father, I trust that you will provide me with the healing remedies my body needs in order to function with boundless energy and suppleness. I was made in your image, and I decree and declare I am strong and healthy. In Jesus's name, amen.

---

[*] "Physical Activity Helps Prevent Chronic Diseases," Centers for Disease Control and Prevention, May 8, 2023, https://www.cdc.gov/chronicdisease/index.htm#:~:text=CDC%2527s%2520NCCDPHP %2520believes%2520that%2520all,to%2520live%2520their%2520healthiest%2520life.&text=Six% 2520in%2520ten%2520Americans%2520live,stroke%252C%2520cancer%252C%2520or%2520diabetes.

DAY 29
BUILD YOUR TRIBE

"Therefore encourage one another and build one another up, just as you are doing."
1 Thessalonians 5:11

Sweaty, spent, and totally exhausted from 55 minutes in a hot yoga class with temps at 100 degrees, I thought the tough part was over. Not just any yoga class, this included high intensity and continuous movement.

"Bring your body into a camel pose," the instructor challenged. For non-yogis, just know, this movement is tough. From a kneeling position, reach back and try to touch your heels. Ouch!

"From camel pose, wheel through a full backbend." She demonstrated flawlessly, while most of the class sighed.

"There's no way I can do that," I admitted.

"You're Shemane Nugent," the instructor declared in front of the whole class. "You're tough as nails."

I was embarrassed, but now I had to at least try.

To go from camel pose to wheel requires passing through a blind spot. I had to trust that when I arched my back further and reached over my head toward the floor, somehow I could land in a perfect backbend. In my mind, I was a flexible teenager. In reality, my muscles and bones had been around for more than five decades.

That's when my friend appeared at my side. "I got you," she said, and wrapped a supportive arm under my back. Together, we did it!

Having a good friend is like having a secret weapon you didn't know you needed. They celebrate your wins and stand by you through difficult times. They can also encourage self-care. Who doesn't love a spa day with a bestie?

Proclaiming intentions to a family member, friend, or on social media is effective to keep us on track, too. Having accountability provides incentive to keep us moving toward accomplishing goals.

When you build your tribe, you may be surprised at who becomes a strong member of your community. My best friend Nancy and I met in junior high school. We both liked a boy who was the playa in our school. One week, he liked Nancy, and the next week he liked me. Nancy was a top tennis athlete and could kick my butt if she wanted to. I was scared of her.

We were on a school ski trip, and wouldn't you know it, Nancy and I showed up with the same ski outfit. I did everything I could to avoid her. She was waiting in line on the opposite side of the chairlift. As we moved closer to the beginning of the line, I saw that Nancy would be sitting with me. This was it. I was sure she would push me off the chairlift.

Eventually, we started talking and realized that this boy really wasn't a great boyfriend at all. And we discovered we had a lot in common. Forty years later, we talk on the phone at least once a day, and Nancy is my son's godmother. I'm forever grateful for my BFF and love having someone with whom I can share my roller-coaster ride of life.

CREATE A SUPPORTIVE COMMUNITY

Having a few people with whom you can share your innermost thoughts, complain about your job or spouse, and who will lift you up during troubling times is one of the best things you can do to stay happy and healthy. Someone outside your immediate family who knows and loves you can be a great source of advice, too. Knowing that you can pick up the phone and call a trustworthy friend who will be there for you in good times and bad can add years to your life.

I still keep in touch with friends I had in high school and college. They know my backstory and I know theirs. We may see one another only every few years, but it always feels comfortable and cozy to catch up. Recalling memorable events can stimulate brain activity, increase oxygen intake due to laughter, and increase feel-good endorphins. The result is a more calm and relaxed feeling.

The emotional and physical value of a vibrant social life is even more important as you age. Friendships often wane as elderly people isolate themselves or when friends die. According to many studies, social interaction can stave off dementia and Alzheimer's and increase life expectancy. Human beings are social creatures. It's natural to want to spend time with others who support and uplift us.

According to a study published in PLoS Medicine, social ties can significantly increase chances of survival.[*] In other words, surround yourself with family and friends who are supportive of your goals. Check in regularly to keep them up to date on your progress.

Even better, create a tribe of folks who will travel the journey to better health with you. We are far more apt to walk each day when meeting a buddy who walks with us. Additionally, we will go faster and farther when working out with a friend. That's why going to a gym and taking classes with other people who are doing the same thing inspire us to make progress.

---

[*] Julianne Holt-Lunstad, Timothy B. Smith, and J. Bradley Layton, "Social Relationships and Mortality Risk: A Meta-Analytic Review," PLOS Medicine, July 27, 2010, https://journals.plos.org/plosmedicine /article?id=10.1371%2Fjournal.pmed.1000316#:~:text=Data%2520across%2520308%252C849%25 20individuals%252C%2520followed,poor%2520or%2520insufficient%2520social%2520relationships.

You are not the only one in your circle who wants to make changes and improvements in your life. Look for people to encourage and who will encourage you at your church, in your friendship circle, online, and in your neighborhood.

MOVE FORWARD

Who can you connect with so you can serve as accountability for one another on the way to accomplishing your goals? How can you commit to supporting them, as well?

PRAYER

Heavenly Father, I'm blessed to have such an amazing group of friends and family. Please continue to bring spirit-filled sisters into my world so that we can encourage and motivate each other. In Jesus's name, amen.

DAY 30
FOOD SWAPS

"Fear not, for I am with you; be not dismayed, for I am your God; I will strengthen you, I will help you, I will uphold you with my righteous right hand." Isaiah 41:10

It was September of 1980 when I walked into my college dormitory cafeteria for the first time. Large pans of cheesy lasagna, meatloaf, golden baked chicken, sweet corn casserole, green bean casserole, mashed potatoes, gravy, soft aromatic bread, cherry pie, chocolate chip cookies, and unlimited self-serve ice cream drew me like a magnet. Three times a day—breakfast, lunch, and dinner—there was a smorgasbord of enticing foods and I could have seconds or thirds.

By December, I couldn't zip my jeans. Two months later, in February of 1981, I officially joined the freshman fifteen club—you know, that unofficial term for college students who pack on an extra fifteen pounds in the first year. This isn't a club you want to join.

But I had a plan. To lose the weight I'd gained my first year in college, I took the extreme opposite approach. Instead of eating everything in sight, I didn't eat at all.

Of course, the results were not impressive. Eventually, I learned that instead of going to the extremes—feasting without restraint or self-inflicted malnutrition—there is a way to find a balanced compromise. By swapping non-essential, superfluous foods with vitamin-packed nourishment, I now avoid empty calorie, nutritionally void food. I'm able to shed pounds or maintain my weight and cultivate a healthier lifestyle.

I developed a system that gives me options to savor the food I love without remorse.

THE PLAN

1. **Commit.** Strike a deal with yourself to eat at least 80 percent whole, God-created food, not man-made, processed foods with preservatives like monosodium glutamate. The downside is you'll spend more time in the kitchen prepping and cooking, but you can focus on the positives. While preparing your own food you can listen to a podcast or call a friend. Spend time with God and pray that your food will bring health and healing.

2. **Choose your weapon.** There are many dietary regimens, so discover what works for you, such as paleo, carnivore, or vegan programs. Proteins like chicken, fish, beef, venison, legumes, or soybeans will keep you feeling full and satisfied longer and

are necessary for building strength, hormone function, healthy hair, and energy production. Plan meals around proteins.

3. **Portion control.** While you can certainly weigh food precisely, most people quickly give up on that step. One rule that's easy to remember is sticking to portions that are approximately the size of your palm—not including the fingers.

4. **Salt it.** If you've been raised to finish the food on your plate, it's difficult to deviate from that custom. We don't want to waste food anyway, right? When you reach the point where you're approximately 70 percent full, sprinkle a generous amount of salt over the remainder of the food. That way you're less likely to eat it.

5. **Pick your battles.** If you know you're going to want dessert, skip the bread and butter. Pass up the whipped cream on your frozen mocha latte to save a hundred empty calories.

6. **Prayer and fasting.** When you realize that certain foods or undesirable behaviors wield influence on you, ask God to intervene. "Which one of you, if his son asks him for bread, will give him a stone? Or if he asks for a fish, will give him a serpent? If you then, who are evil, know how to give good gifts to your children, how much more will your Father who is in heaven give good things to those who ask him!" Matthew 7:9–11.

SWAP

- Bread and butter—cheese and crackers
- Frozen margarita—club soda or spritzer with frozen fruit
- Chips and salsa—sliced vegetables with hummus
- Cookies and cake—peanut butter protein balls (See Recipes, page 123.)
- Soda—sparkling water with fruit and herbs
- Processed foods—whole foods
- Coffee creamer—half-and-half (without carrageenan)
- Dessert after dinner—a couple of dark chocolate squares
- Gravy—olive oil and spices
- Refined sugar—natural sweeteners like honey, monk fruit, stevia, applesauce, or dates
- White rice—brown rice
- White flour—whole wheat, almond, oat, chickpea, spelt, or rice flour
- Canola or vegetable oil—avocado or extra virgin olive oil
- Tortillas—lettuce wraps
- Pizza crust—cauliflower crust
- Genetically modified food—locally farmed food grown outdoors in direct sunlight withouthormones, antibiotics, or vaccines

One of the best ways to avoid overindulging and anxiety around mealtimes is to swap the guilt and stress for prayer and self-care. Pause and take a moment to think about what is happening in your body and where you feel tension. Is your heart rate elevated? Shoulders tense? Remove yourself from the environment, go for a walk, inhale deeply, and talk to God. "Casting all your anxieties on him, because he cares for you," 1 Peter 5:7. The act of praying can be incredibly calming and provide a sense of comfort and inner peace. God wants us to express our anxieties and worries. "And which of you by being anxious can add a single hour to his span of life?" Luke 12:25.

Get plenty of exercise. Regular physical activity releases endorphins and hormones like cortisol and adrenaline that are produced in response to stress and anxiety. Exercise can help improve your moods and even reduce symptoms of depression.

Avoid excessive alcohol. Oftentimes that second glass of wine or beer can lead to poor nutritional choices. Unwittingly, while sipping too much, your inhibitions are lowered. Your brain might trick you into thinking you're hungry or thirsty. You may be tempted to indulge in more carbohydrate-rich or salty food.

MOVE FORWARD

Prepare ahead. When you attend a potentially tense social gathering, decide ahead of time what food you will eat and what you will not eat. Know before going what you will drink and what you will not. This alleviates decision fatigue and allows clarity for being in the situation.

PRAYER

Heavenly Father, forgive me for not putting you at the center of my world and for relying on earthly pleasures like food and alcohol to fill me, calm me, and distract me. Send your Holy Spirit to fill the void that lies within me and to comfort me. Lead me not into temptation. I trust you and know I can do all things through you, God. In Jesus's name, amen.

REIMAGINE AGING

"Gray hair is a crown of glory; it is gained in a righteous life." Proverbs 16:31

My husband, rocker Ted Nugent, asked me to dance onstage at a concert in front of twenty thousand people. Problem was, I was nearly fifty years old. *Why hadn't he asked me when I was thirty or even forty?*

Had it not been for my previous life-threatening illness, I don't think I would have agreed to bust a move onstage at a rock 'n' roll concert while also suffering from arthritis. Wasn't I too old? I continued to dance at Ted's concerts on stage in front of thousands (50,000 at the Swedish Rock Fest) until I was fifty-two. Although he continued to ask me to salsa onstage during *Stranglehold*, I decided to bow out gracefully and move on to something else.

Similarly, Sister Madonna Buder, a Roman Catholic nun, took up running when she was forty-eight. Dubbed the Iron Nun for competing in Ironman triathlons and breaking records at age eighty-six, Sister Madonna's tenacity, courage, and strength proved that aging with health, vitality, and grace is possible.

My grandmother became Ms. Senior Michigan when she was eighty-nine. Gram was a popular entertainer, playing the keyboard and belting out tunes like Ella Fitzgerald at nightclubs until her early nineties. President George Bush went skydiving when he was ninety years old.

Can we *redefine* misconceptions about the elderly population? If you *reframe* your mindset and shift your perspective, you will begin to see a bright future with unlimited potential.

Aging gracefully is the practice of looking at growing old as an amazing gift, sparked with excitement. Rather than disdain brown spots, changes in our skin, and getting up in the night to use the bathroom, *reimagine* the concept of aging as the greatest, most exhilarating, and sought-after experience of our lives. The dark trials and tribulations we've experienced provide insight and wisdom. People who suffered tragic losses or survived life-threatening illness say those difficult times helped them appreciate the gift of life and take more chances. Wrinkles are worthy of honor, appreciation, and respect, especially when the longer we live, the greater we live.

REIMAGINE AGING

Does aging gracefully mean you can do the splits when you're seventy years old? Start a new business? As we age, we can give ourselves permission to wear comfortable shoes, run a marathon, *and* get a senior discount at the restaurant all in the same day. We simply *reframe* what we thought we knew about aging.

Most likely you've worked hard, raised kids, and now you're exhausted. Or maybe you're complacent. Perhaps you feel as though you're too old to start something new. What has the Holy Spirit been nudging you to do? "Having gifts that differ according to the grace given to us, let us use them: if prophecy, in proportion to our faith; if service, in our serving; the one who teaches, in his teaching; the one who exhorts, in his exhortation; the one who contributes, in generosity; the one who leads, with zeal; the one who does acts of mercy, with cheerfulness," Romans 12:6–8.

Finding joy in life is a significant aspect of aging gracefully. If you've spent thirty or forty exhausting years creating habits and patterns, the concept of change is daunting. If you've lived your life putting the needs of others before your own, changing your mindset can be a challenge, *if you let it*. Practice gratitude for a sunny day, a child's laugh, or snuggling with a pet. Joyfulness replaces feelings of overwhelm.

Instead of telling yourself you're not good enough, smart enough, or young enough, replace those negative thoughts with positive affirmations.

- *I'm not smart enough* can become *I'll learn what I need to know.*
- Substitute *I don't know where to start* for *I'll make a plan and do one small thing each day.*
- Conquer frustration with *I will allow myself time to try a new hobby.*
- Relieve stress with *I may make mistakes and have setbacks, but I will stay committed.*
- Give yourself grace with *the results of a new diet and exercise program may not happen overnight. I will be patient.*

If the twentieth year of the twenty-first century showed us anything, it's that everything can change in the blink of an eye. In a few short months, we went from planning Spring Break to prepping for quarantine. Weddings, funerals, graduations, and even simple barbecues were postponed. Finding toilet paper on grocery store shelves was equivalent to winning the lottery. A new fashion trend emerged as millennials in lockdown dyed their hair gray. Suddenly, going gray was *en vogue*.

Reports indicated that between 2015 and 2050, the proportion of the world's population over sixty years old will nearly double, from 12 percent to 22 percent.[*] Let's showcase mountain climbers in their eighties and super model seventy-year-olds. Those in our fifties, sixties,

---

[*] "Ageing and Health," World Health Organization, October 1, 2022, https://www.who.int/news-room/fact-sheets/detail/ageing-and-health#:~:text=The%2520pace%2520of%2520population%2520ageing,from%252012%2525%2520to%252022%2525.

seventies, and beyond understand the joy of simple things including good health, a beautiful sunset, and sleeping through the night.

During the second half of life, as children leave home and need less attention, we can reset our internal clocks and add a few precious moments of "me time." Those extra sixty minutes feel almost like a vacation. You don't have to rush. You can sleep a little extra, get more work done, or take a longer bath. With a reframe of our mindset, our own personal needs are given a priority. Recall those childhood dreams and goals. Focus on minding your own good health. Are there extra pounds to release? Habits to change?

But we're older, our bones ache, and we cannot physically do what we used to do. How do we reclaim that uninhibited, childlike joy for life without a trip to the emergency room for broken bones? What do we want to do with the rest of our lives? How do we reimagine, redefine, and reframe our thoughts, physical bodies, and our spirits?

We can work with what we have, what we enjoy, and what's available.

- What are your passions, talents, and skills? Think about those things you liked to do as a kid.
- What are your gifts and talents?

If you struggle with answering these questions, ask friends or family members. Oftentimes, we fail to see ourselves the way others see us. Maybe you're good at organizing, or you have a knack for numbers. Do you enjoy writing, jewelry-making, collecting, or researching family history?

People who are close to you might be able to help you see yourself in a different light. Together, you can visualize how the second half of your lives could turn out if you had the good health and energy to accomplish your goals. It's important to be realistic. The window may be closed for winning a gold medal at the Olympics, but why not the Senior Olympics?

Aging gracefully is not just about the way we look. It's about improving and enhancing the way we think, feel, and act. Sometimes a subtle shift can make a huge difference. Or perhaps a bold and brave move is necessary, like physically removing obstacles or spending less time with people and environments that prevent you from living a happier life. Exchanging a frustrating, dead-end job with an occupation about which you're excited may prove fulfilling. Distancing or removing a toxic person from your life can give a fresh perspective about how the relationship can move forward with love and joy rather than angst and anger. A glimmer of hope can transform doubt and spark a more positive outlook.

Allow yourself to *redefine* what aging means to you, take action to *reframe* your approach, and you can *reawaken* your body, mind, and spirit. Make appointments with yourself to exercise and to learn a new hobby or skill. Just as you wouldn't miss a doctor appointment—especially one for your kids—write *Me Time* into your schedule. Get involved in a book club, a tech class, or the Chamber of Commerce. Create a bucket list of activities and try one each month.

Thinking with your mind and physically doing something with your body improves those neurological pathways. Communicating with like-minded people buoys your spirits and confidence. Give yourself grace.

When I consider Sister Madonna Buda or my grandmother, I see lives well-lived. Being an octogenarian didn't stop them from running marathons or entertaining at nightclubs.

MOVE FORWARD

How can you *reimagine* new possibilities for the rest of your life? What are your deepest hopes and dreams? Take a few minutes to create a bucket list for new adventures.

PRAYER

Heavenly father, I come to you, humbled and grateful. You know every gray hair on my head, and you still love me. Help me to see myself through your eyes and know that I am worthy. Let me be comforted and anchored in your peace and protection. Give me strength and courage to reimagine my life as I age like fine wine. Let me understand your will for my life. In Jesus's name, amen.

DAY 32
ALLERGIES

"For everything created by God is good, and nothing is to be rejected if it is received with thanksgiving." 1 Timothy 4:4

I f you've been reading these devotions in order, you know a little about how toxic mold in our home almost killed me, but there's more I want to share with you about that experience. As a group fitness instructor since 1980, I've appeared in exercise videos and cable TV shows. I know my body, and I know when something doesn't feel right. Around 2002, I began to have flu-like symptoms and debilitating migraines.

I became constantly tired and hadn't had a good night's sleep in years. Ten minutes into the exercise classes I instructed, I couldn't get enough air, and I was scared. Something was terribly wrong but I couldn't figure it out.

Then my son, Rocco, developed constant allergies, anemia, and severe asthma. My husband had symptoms similar to mine. Neither of us could sleep. We had short-term memory loss, achy joints, and flu-like symptoms.

Doctors told us we were too busy, which was true, so we ignored the blatant message our bodies were sending and chalked it up to being overworked. One doctor told me I might be too healthy and I should eat more fast food.

The light bulb moment came when we traveled to London. The three of us slept like babies and felt great. When we returned home, sleep eluded us as our bodies shook as if being slowly electrified.

We discovered our house, once featured on MTV Cribs, was the cause of this mysterious sickness. Toxic mold had been secretly growing between the walls and circulated through the house by the air system until our home became a slow killer. A toxicologist concluded that Ted and I had four types of mold in our blood and diagnosed me with pre-emphysema.

We left our beloved home, a beautiful, five-thousand-square-foot house that stood majestically overlooking a lake with ducks and geese—a place where we had made so many beautiful memories. We walked out with the clothes on our backs, and then we got rid of them.

YOUR BODY'S SIGNALS

It doesn't matter if you live in Antarctica or Florida, if you have a porous substance, lack of ventilation, and water infiltration, you will have deadly toxic mold contamination. Some people react more strongly to mold than others. In the same way, people have allergic reactions to all kinds of things from peanuts to pollen. According to the Centers for Disease Control and Prevention, allergies are the sixth leading cause of chronic illness in the United States.[*]

Have you been ignoring minor or major aches and pains? Is your body trying to tell you something? Allergy symptoms are your body's signal to you that something in your life needs to be addressed. Something is compromising your health. Unfortunately, I didn't listen to my body and became deathly ill. I couldn't walk up a flight of stairs if my life depended on it. I thought my days of teaching group fitness classes were over. I was dying.

Fortunately, the human body has an amazing ability to heal, and after a year of detoxifying my body, I regained my health. I am now an International Zumba® Fitness Presenter and Instructor, sharing my passion for healthy living.

When someone experiences a perpetual runny nose, itchy eyes or skin, headache, rash, fatigue, and foggy brain, it could be your body telling you there is an allergen present. Not everyone is allergic to the same things. What bothers one person will have no effect on another. The key is to diagnose and take steps to alleviate the problem. Mold is bad for everyone. Others are sensitive to foods, trees, and animal dander. One friend had her preschooler tested and found the child was sensitive to dust. She removed the carpet and decor items that collected and held dust in the child's room and the symptoms became manageable.

For those living with allergens, their body is constantly on high alert, constantly fighting invaders that are harmful. The exhausted immune system becomes compromised and secondary issues complicate an already strained system.

A helpful two-pronged approach is to remove the allergen while simultaneously boosting the immune system. Do research and meet with professionals in the field who can help you craft a plan toward optimum health.

MOVE FORWARD

If you have symptoms you've been ignoring, become a sleuth for better health. Research natural cures for your symptoms on the Internet. Talk to multiple doctors. These ailments could be something serious.

PRAYER

I declare a miracle healing, oh Lord! I rebuke the spirit of infirmity! Let the light of Jesus surround me, comfort me, and restore my health. You have called me to do great things. For that, I need a fit and sound body, mind, and spirit. In Jesus's name, amen.

---

[*] "Facts and Stats—50 Million Americans Have Allergies: Acaai Patient," ACAAI Public Website, June 28, 2023, https://acaai.org/allergies/allergies-101/facts-stats/.

RADICAL REST

"In peace I will both lie down and sleep;
for you alone, O Lord, make me dwell in safety." Psalm 4:8

It was two o'clock in the morning when I first felt it. Lying in bed, my legs started vibrating under the sheets. Certain there was something—maybe a mouse!—in the bed, I screamed, woke my husband, and pulled off the sheets so violently that I knocked over a lamp. Dazed, delirious, and ready to go into combat mode, my husband asked if I heard a noise outside. "No! There's a mouse or something in the mattress!" I yelled.

There wasn't.

Ted was on hiatus from his concert tours. Our *New York Times* bestselling wild game cookbook, *Kill It & Grill It*, had recently released. In three hours we had to leave the house and fly to New York City, where a dozen television and radio interviews were scheduled for us to promote our book. We needed a good night's sleep to begin the book tour looking rested and healthy. Instead, our bloodshot and hooded eyes made us look twice our age.

For more than a year, neither of us could sleep well. We chalked it up to being overworked and over-scheduled. Instead of six to eight hours of rest, we rock and rolled our way to dawn each night, bleary eyed and exhausted the next day.

The mouse in our bed turned out to be a something called Restless Leg Syndrome, mainly caused by pregnancy, obesity, or smoking. None of which applied to us. After completely dismantling the sheets, the mattress, and a failed but intense search for that darn mouse, we tried to fall back asleep. The digital alarm clock flipped from two o'clock to three o'clock, and then it was four-thirty. Time to awake! With heavy legs and bloodshot eyes, we headed to the airport.

SWEET SLEEP

According to the American Sleep Association, 50 to 70 million US adults have a sleep disorder.[*] Getting enough sleep is a vital, irreplaceable aspect of being healthy. Adequate sleep

---

[*] "Sleep Health," National Heart Lung and Blood Institute, accessed April 4, 2024, https://www.nhlbi.nih .gov/health-topics/education-and-awareness/sleep-health#:~:text=About%252050%2520to%252070 %2520million,need%2520to%2520protect%2520their%2520health.

improves our appearance and how we feel and function emotionally, mentally, physically, and spiritually.

Emotionally, we are less fragile when rested. Mentally, good sleep allows us to think with clarity and make better decisions. Physically, excellent shut-eye makes us better coordinated and less prone to accidents. Spiritually, we are more discerning of God's voice and guidance when our mind is clear of the fog that settles over a brain that has not slept well.

Sleep boosts immune function and sharpens memory. Many are surprised to see their metabolism and weight settle into healthy parameters once the body gets adequate sleep. The older I get, the more I appreciate a successful slumber. But many factors can make getting good, restful sleep difficult.

According to the International Labor Organization, Americans work 137 more hours per year than Japanese workers, 260 more hours per year than British workers, and 499 more hours per year than French workers. A lack of sleep has been compared with being intoxicated. "Losing four hours of sleep is comparable to drinking a six-pack of beer," says Tom Rath, author of the *New York Times* bestselling book, *Eat Move Sleep*.

The National Sleep Foundation recommends that adults aim for seven to nine hours of sleep per night for optimal health. Facilitate radical rest for health and well-being by creating an uncompromising self-care routine to rejuvenate your mind, body, and spirit. To improve your sleep:

1. Try organic bedding, mattresses, and pillows
2. Move electrical appliances including alarm clocks at least seven feet from your bed
3. Avoid cell phones, computer use, and other screen devices at least two hours before bedtime
4. Stop caffeinated drinks eight hours before bedtime
5. Take a few minutes to meditate, relax, pray, and stretch before bed
6. Make sure your bed and pillows are clean and comfortable
7. Journal for five minutes, listing three things you are thankful for and three things to do the next day. Empty these on paper so your mind is free to relax.

Sometimes we overthink problems causing our brain to be on a constantly repeating soundtrack. When we don't sleep well, we're tired, have brain fog, and are less productive the next day. Taking prescription drugs to stay awake or go to sleep adds chemicals to your body and contributes to lethargy the next day. Highly caffeinated drinks designed to keep you awake are hard on the body and heart.

Create a bedtime routine that includes the things listed above to encourage beneficial sleep.

REST YOUR MIND

Close your eyes, put your hand on your chest, and feel your heartbeat. Focus on slowing your breath. Beginning with your forehead and moving to your toes, relax every part of your body. Imagine every cell in your body is operating at its utmost potential. Envision every muscle and bone healthy and strong. Bring your awareness to your breath. Pretend you're breathing through a straw slowly. Inhale to the count of ten and exhale slowly. Feel your heartbeat slow.

Studies show we can reduce stress, lower blood pressure, lower the risk of heart attacks and strokes, and diminish anxiety by being still and calming our bodies and minds. Meditation helps the mind find a happy ground where it's not working so hard and spinning out of control. Stillness helps control anxious and negative thoughts.

We live in a world that exposes us to way too much information. Take a look at network or cable news programs; watch the constant ticker tape running with breaking news stories while the newscaster is interjecting information. Note the station logo in the corner and the backdrop of moving designs. Unfortunately, we have become used to information overload. Our bodies, minds, spirits, and emotions crave stillness. In the quiet we listen to the messages our bodies are communicating.

Ever walk into a room and wonder why you're there? We're a nation—a world—of over-achievers; we do too much and think too much.

Do you notice that your mind becomes too busy and you tend to overthink things? Be still and calm your many minds. When sleep is elusive because your many minds are moving fast, use the technique described above. After your bedtime routine, get comfortable in bed. Slow your breathing and relax each place in your body beginning at your head and making your way to your toes. Take another deep breath and sink deeply into the mattress.

MOVE FORWARD

Choose something from the list to incorporate into your bedtime routine today. Then select another item until the list becomes a regular habit.

PRAYER

Father, I come to you in need of good slumber. Matthew 11:28 says, "Come to me, all who labor and are heavy laden, and I will give you rest." I surrender my troubles to you, Lord. If it be your will, let me sleep peacefully tonight and wake feeling rested. Breathe new life into my weary bones. In Jesus's name, amen.

DAY 34
BOUNDARIES & STRESS

"Keep your heart with all vigilance, for from it flow the springs of life." Proverbs 4:23

We decided to have a girls-night-in. Everyone brought something to eat or drink and we caught up on the latest in each other's lives. One friend showed up in her pajamas, and that was awesome! As the Texas sun set overlooking our magnificent Serengeti field, we took off our shoes, pulled up our knees, and relaxed on comfy patio furniture near a gas fireplace.

Laughter was prevalent and welcomed. Smiles galore, I remember thinking we need to do this more often. Sharing laughter with others strengthens our social support system and provides a sense of belonging. It triggers the release of neurotransmitters that counter stress.

Many of us are just too serious. We seldom have laugh-out-loud fun. Play is the antithesis to stress and vital for self-care. Playtime helps us physically and mentally by allowing us to exercise and be creative. Our imagination can be stimulated through a childlike recess. Physical exercise can release endorphins that create a feeling of euphoria, assuaging the ravages of stress on our minds and bodies. These hormones are also used to reduce inflammation and block pain. On top of it all, having fun burns calories, keeps us young, and helps us to temporarily ignore our troubles.

When my son, Rocco, was growing up, I was the parent on her knees crawling through the play centers. Jumping on the trampoline and skiing with my grandkids makes me grateful to have a strong and still energetic body.

Purposely schedule play into each day. Even a few minutes can have a significant impact on your well-being. Here are a few things you can do to play today:

- Turn on music and dance
- Go to a park and climb on the monkey bars
- Play with your dog
- Ride a bike
- Jump on a trampoline

BOUNDARIES

When play is absent from our life, it can also signify a lack of boundaries. Too much work and worry leads to an unbalanced and unhealthy life and curtails longevity. Having boundaries is synonymous with self-care. We can allow negative situations to wear out our patience, leaving us drained and exhausted. There are people in all of our lives who siphon the positive feeling from us and zap our strength. Try as we might, we can't always avoid these energy vampires.

Rocco and I were in an elevator when a man rushed in as the doors closed. His heavy breathing and frantic demeanor indicated he was in a rush and had someplace else to be. The problem was, Rocco and I were stuck in a small space with him and his toxic energy. He thumped the button repeatedly, as if hitting it faster and harder would get us to the tenth floor more quickly. When he finally exited, Rocco and I looked at each other with confusion and exhaustion etched into our faces. Have you experienced something similar when someone else's bad vibes cause your typically happy demeanor to become tainted?

I believe this is spiritual warfare. "The thief comes only to steal and kill and destroy. I came that they may have life and have it abundantly," John 10:10. Jesus dealt with energy vampires, too. People were never satisfied with his answers and challenged him. "The Pharisees came and began to argue with him, seeking from him a sign from heaven to test him," Mark 8:11.

When I feel that toxic energy is stealing my peace of mind, I take a deep breath and say a silent prayer that God will send His warring angels to protect me from the evil one. I may even go into the bathroom and rebuke Satan. It could get loud, and if you ever hear me shouting in a public restroom, that's most likely what's going on. I envision God's wings wrapped around me.

People cannot steal your happiness unless you let them. But darn. Some are really good at taunting you, pushing your buttons, and getting an unsavory reaction.

Are there any energy vampires in your life? What proactive steps can you take to prevent your energy from being hijacked?

The opposite of burnout is found in radical rest. Boundaries set the context for peace, rest, and serenity. The American Psychological Association suggests that establishing healthy boundaries can reduce stress and improve overall well-being.[*]

We are all busy, but if you only live your life to please others, fulfill responsibilities, and work, you may become resentful and may not be living God's dream for you. "Come to me, all who labor and are heavy laden, and I will give you rest," Matthew 11:28.

Before diving into someone else's conflict, ask yourself:

- In the past, does this person seem to be surrounded with an abundance of tribulations?

---

[*]   Tori DeAngelis, "Boundary Watch," American Psychological Association, November 2009, https://www .apa.org/gradpsych/2009/11/boundary.

- Do they consistently make bad choices that create unfortunate outcomes?
- Do they ignore intelligent advice?
- Do they surround themselves with an unhealthy environment such as excessive smoking, drinking, gambling, or something similar?

As we dig ourselves deeper into the helping hole, we can wind up unable to find a way out for ourselves, especially if we are emotionally tied to that person as a close friend or family member. Of course, there are definitely times in all of our lives when we need the guidance of people we trust to have our backs in good times and bad.

When bad vibes are more prevalent than good ones, the best approach is to save yourself and bow out of the battle gracefully. Having boundaries with people who seem to be surrounded by a dizzying level of chaos is a healthier choice.

MOVE FORWARD

What did you do for your playtime today? Learn to say "no" to obligations that aren't in your best interest and to people who don't make you feel like sunshine. If saying no is a challenge, instead say, "I will get back to you about that." Take 24 hours to pray about it, consider your schedule, and make a smart decision about whether that particular obligation aligns with your goals for improved health and lifestyle. When something is not a fit, respond with, "Thank you for asking, but I have to pass."

PRAYER

Father, my eyes are fixed on you today. Help me to focus on your word instead of anyone else who might steal my joy. I need your help, Father, to avoid the pitfalls of the enemy who tries to drag me down and prevent me from experiencing your peace. In loving praise, amen.

NATURE AS HEALER

BY TED NUGENT

"The heavens declare the glory of God, and the sky above proclaims his handiwork. Day to day pours out speech, and night to night reveals knowledge. There is no speech, nor are there words, whose voice is not heard. Their voice goes out through all the earth, and their words to the end of the world." Psalm 19:1–4

I hadn't seen a buck in three days. Hadn't taken a shot at a deer in over a week. But I could feel the smile on my face. After all, it's not like I was short on backstraps.

The season was only two weeks old and I had made wonderful arrows on two fat yearling does and a handsome butterball forked horn buck, so the sacred straps were mounting up nicely. Much more importantly, I was hunting, baby. Celebrating my fifty-eighth amazing season in the American deerwoods, trusty bow and arrows in hand, spirit soaring in my heart, and wild ground pulsing underfoot. It just doesn't get any better than that.

It all started back in the 1940s for the Nugent tribe. My dad had just returned from the hellfire war against the evil Japanese Empire and the demonic Nazi stormtroopers. He landed home in this great country after watching so many heroes of the US Military warriors sacrifice everything for freedom. Dad felt weary and beat, in desperate need of spiritual cleansing and American Dream recreation. It was a terrible cross to bear for the brave men and women who gave so much as good warred over evil in WWII and Korea. He, like his Blood Brothers, needed rest.

Thankfully, great men like Fred Bear in Michigan and Roy Case in Wisconsin were rediscovering the joys of the mystical flight of the arrow, and returning to a pure, aboriginal connection with the good Mother Earth through the incredible challenge of hunting with the bow and arrow.

Ishi, the last Yahi Indian of Northern California, had recently passed this deeply spiritual lifestyle to Saxon Pope and Art Young and an ever-growing cadre of hardcore, dedicated sporters. The demands for a higher level of awareness through bowhunting brought to them a deeper relationship with nature. Harvested forests across North America were exploding into ideal deer habitat. In this target-rich environment came the rebirth for bowhunting, and my dad, Warren Henry Nugent, got the fire.

I remember our family excursions up North each October like they were yesterday. That smell, those colors, the intensity of big game dreams, the silent walks in the cathedral of the big timber, those mesmerizing, feathered arrows, the grace of a bent bow. The call of the wild was a glorious force to reckon with, and I was hooked, mind, body, spirit, and soul. Every moment on the hunt simply made me feel more alive. I couldn't get enough of it. God made me a hunter.

My father is gone now. Fred and Roy and most of the founding fathers of this great archery hunting lifestyle are in the wind when I return to the sacred hunting grounds of my youth. Now I share these precious moments and vital sensations with my children, my wife, and brothers and sisters and family and friends. The experience is more desirable, more enjoyable, and more intense now than ever in all of my fifty-nine years.

I learned that the backstraps will come if I follow nature's lead. I practice in order to kill game, and I will eventually. But it is the healing power of nature that ultimately lures me back. Like my hunting friends and Blood Brothers, I crave that road less traveled. I live for a sunrise and a birdsong. I revel in the thunder of a drumming grouse, the chattering of a bushy-tail limbrat. The call of brother crow and raven. I stand in awe of the miraculous wildlife that brings joy, challenge, and protein.

Surely, hunting is the last perfect touch with God's tooth, fang, and claw creation. I look to the heavens in humble servitude to God's laws of conservation and stewardship. I kill to eat and bring balance and health to the sacred land that fuels my family's life. I consume with reverence the miraculous renewable resources with which we are blessed. I serve with a smile and a predator heartbeat. My soul is cleansed with the spirit of the wild each and every time I go back, back where I belong.

There is very little perfection that mankind can claim to be a part of in the modern world. Nurturing, protecting, and providing for our families are certainly perfect functions of the heart. And so is hunting, fishing, trapping, and giving back to the land.

The beast will come. I will dedicate myself to be the best reasoning predator that I can be. The gift of sacred flesh will come my way. I will pick a spot, and if I pray, I will kill the beast. Reverence will be given for the gift, and the circle will go unbroken. It is the way. It is life. It is death. It is perfect. The beast is dead, long live the beast. And he will heal me forevermore.

MOVE FORWARD

Take a walk outside without your phone. Make a mental note of what you see, hear, and smell. Try to do this anytime you're feeling the least bit stressed or overwhelmed.

PRAYER

God, I thank you for the amazing gifts of nature: the singing birds, the gentle whispering of leaves as they sway in the wind, and how being immersed in the great outdoors brings me calm and peace. Speak to me, Father, every time I step outside. Hear my voice and allow me to hear yours. In Jesus's mighty name, amen.

DAY 36
CHARITY

"If you pour yourself out for the hungry and satisfy the desire of the afflicted, then shall your light rise in the darkness and your gloom be as the noonday." Isaiah 58:10

Taking the focus off myself and putting it on others has always lifted me from the deepest, darkest depths of despair.

In 2004, Ted, Rocco, and I visited veterans at Brooke Army Medical Center in San Antonio. We went from room to room, visiting severely injured soldiers. The sights were worse than any Hollywood movie could depict. Ted played his guitar and entertained the troops in a rehab room. A young man who had suffered serious burns all over his body was strapped onto a bed. He moaned while his limbs were stretched to encourage new skin to grow.

As we ascended to higher floors, the wounds seemed to get worse. Though half her face had been maimed, a beautiful, dark-haired woman smiled wide and bright as she talked about recovering quickly and rejoining her fellow soldiers.

A nineteen-year-old corporal John Chrzanowski had been brought in the night before we arrived. Wrapped from head to toe like a mummy, he had been burned all over his body. To minimize the chance for infection, his visitors were kept to a minimum. Ted scrubbed, put on a face mask and gown, and went to talk with John.

Rocco and I stood outside with John's mother. I had no idea what to say to her. How could any words bring her comfort?

"Do you need anything?" I asked. "Can I do anything for you?"

"My son is an outdoorsman." She lifted her chin. "I can't imagine him recovering without being able to get outside."

Glancing about I noticed there was no patio at BAMC to shelter burned and wounded veterans from direct sunlight.

I had zero experience with fundraising and no idea how I would do it, but I told Nancy I'd raise the money to build a patio at the center so her son and others could get outside into fresh air but stay out of the sun.

With the help of my husband, Ted, Texas governor Rick Perry, and many others, a beautiful pavilion was created at Brooke Army Medical Center, providing relief to hundreds of deserving and honored American military veterans. That experience prompted me to start Freedom's Angels to help wounded soldiers and their families. We raised money to provide a track chair to a veteran who had lost his legs. Now, he can go to the beach with his family and not worry about the complications of walking with prosthetic legs in the sand.

GET INVOLVED

Ted and I help raise money for several organizations benefiting veterans, children, and animals. One charity placed shelter dogs with veterans suffering from post-traumatic stress. We've hosted children with terminal illnesses at our home. Meeting children stricken by a death warrant is heartbreaking. It's so unfair to them and their families. How dare I complain of having a bad hair day or gaining a few pounds? Those families would prefer to have my problems.

Whenever I have my pity days, I think about people who struggle with much more daunting tribulations, and I get involved. "Whoever is generous to the poor lends to the Lord, and he will repay him for his deed," Proverbs 19:17. One Thanksgiving, Ted, Rocco, and I went to a soup kitchen and served the homeless.

Giving USA reports that Americans gave $449.64 billion to charity in 2019, an increase of 5.1 percent compared to the previous year.[*] Lending a helping hand to others comes in countless forms.

- Give financially to organizations that make a difference
- Volunteer at your local school
- Give your time at a hospital
- Do crafts and make puzzles at a retirement home
- Provide diapers and baby items to pregnancy centers
- Sponsor a student to attend a workshop or college
- Pay for a child to have music lessons or to be on a sports team
- Teach Sunday school so parents can have one hour to sit and be spiritually fed

Most importantly, look around. What will make life better for another? Like John's mother at the BAMC, is someone saying what is needed? Ask the Lord to show you where he wants you to make a difference. Some giving we do ourselves. Sometimes we partner with others because more can be accomplished together.

To be of benefit is a powerful reason to get and stay healthy. Focusing on others provides a sense of purpose and meaning in our lives. Being others-centered reminds us to be

---

[*] "Giving USA 2020: Charitable Giving Showed Solid Growth, Climbing to $449.64 Billion in 2019, One of the Highest Years for Giving on Record: Giving USA," Giving USA | A public service initiative of the Giving Institute, June 17, 2020, https://givingusa.org/giving-usa-2020-charitable-giving-showed -solid-growth-climbing-to-449-64-billion-in-2019-one-of-the-highest-years-for-giving-on-record/.

appreciative of what we have. Coming alongside another is how we hear their story and help carry their burdens. Charity is a deeper way to connect and form a community. Helping others without expectation for repayment brings peace to the soul.

MOVE FORWARD

What can you do to help someone today? This week? This month? How about this year? Using your gifts and talents, in what way can you be of service to a charity organization in your area?

PRAYER

Lord, put in my path someone who needs my help today. Let me take the emphasis off me and my problems and be an example of your good works. I'm ready to serve you and them. In Jesus's name, amen.

DAY 37
MOLD & LYME DISEASE

"When there is a case of leprous disease in a garment, whether a woolen or a linen garment, in warp or woof of linen or wool, or in a skin or in anything made of skin, if the disease is greenish or reddish in the garment, or in the skin or in the warp or the woof or in any article made of skin, it is a case of leprous disease, and it shall be shown to the priest." Leviticus 13:47–49

One day, I offered to bring a hot-from-the-oven batch of my famous, gooey, chocolate chip cookies to Ted and some hunters at our preserve a few miles from our home. But with the onset of a wicked migraine, I telephoned Ted to tell him there would be no homemade treats because I was throwing up from the pain.

When Ted came home later that day, he brought one of his hunting buddies. The last thing I wanted to do was entertain. I had zero energy and had not even brushed my hair.

"Just give me fifteen minutes of your time," Ted's hunting friend said. "I think I can help you."

Ted and I listened as this man described each of our symptoms from joint pain to short-term memory loss.

"Ted, did you tell him all this?" I felt perturbed that my husband would share such personal information.

Ted shook his head. "Just that you had migraines, neither of us could sleep, and we hadn't been feeling well."

How could this casual acquaintance possibly know intimate details about our body aches and ailments?

"Your symptoms," he said, "are eerily similar to those of mold illness."

Each person exposed to toxic mold will have a different experience. As part of my recovery process, I entered an inpatient clinic where I met others who had been impacted by mold. Hunched in his chair, pale and expressionless, a veteran looked as if he'd experienced more than the war. Another woman who had been exposed to mold through the walls in her apartment said she didn't even remember getting to the center.

Toxic mold and Lyme disease can cause devastating health issues. What you need to know about these silent killers is there's not a specific drug to cure the problem. Treating chronic mold exposure is challenging because people have long-term issues after the problem has been remediated. Symptoms of mold exposure can be highly varied and include:

- Allergic reactions
- Breathing issues
- Gastrointestinal problems
- Immunological problems
- Neurological problems
- Pulmonary issues

Functional medicine is the most effective approach for a patient with mold exposure. Looking beyond pharmaceuticals, surgery, chemotherapy, and radiation, this holistic approach considers lifestyle, nutrition, an individual's genomics, and what's going on in the gut. Functional medicine cultivates a program unique for the needs of each unique patient.

Particularly with children, what appears to be allergies can be the body's reaction to mold exposure. Some pediatricians and allergists are recommending patients talk with a mold expert to check for possible exposure in the home. What begins as allergic reactions become worse and create other problems when a body makes more antibodies to compensate for the allergy symptoms.

Chronic fatigue is one of the first signs of a toxigenic exposure to mold, though an allergic response has been widely accepted in the medical community. When exposed to toxic mold, our bodies make an antigen that is excreted through the body to fight the microscopic invader.

But for some individuals, that defense is not enough. Mold toxins attack each person's system differently. Many people can't make antibodies against the toxins and they can't release them. Instead, our fighter cells, which are cytokines, start fighting everything causing inflammation. The cytokines move easily through the blood brain barrier and through organs but are not excreted. The buildup of cytokines causes extreme inflammation that prevents organs from functioning properly and interferes with energy levels.

Teachers and their students experience symptoms when mold has grown in school buildings. Employees who get frequent headaches at work, have difficulty sleeping, trouble remembering, and feel exhausted during the workweek may be reacting to mold in the workplace.

Many molds produce neurotoxins that affect memory. Allergy symptoms, cognitive impairment, headaches, and fatigue are found in settings where people don't know mold is present, or they can see water damage but addressing the problem has been delayed. For individuals with certain genotypes, it is not enough to remove them from the toxins and mold spores. They initially become more ill because the toxins emerge from the biomass around the cells to be excreted with an antioxidant such as glutathione.

LYME

There's a close association between Lyme disease and toxic mold. Lyme causes inflammation in the body and the infected individual may develop a myriad of symptoms from headaches to joint pain.

The interesting connection between Lyme disease and mold illness is that not everyone is affected by these diseases the same way. Both illnesses can mimic other inflammatory maladies like fibromyalgia, chronic fatigue syndrome, and multiple sclerosis.[*] The Lyme spirochete reacts similarly to the mold mycotoxin within the body and can lay dormant for months or years. An infected person might feel better for a period only to have symptoms return, often fueled by stress.

Having Lyme and living in a moldy home is like tossing gasoline onto a fire.

WHAT TO DO

One of the worst situations is when someone feels they're getting sick in their home but doesn't see the visible signs of mold. Symptoms including constant headaches or a runny nose can be explained away with, "It's allergy season" or "I'm just too stressed."

- **Create a game plan.** Make a list of the actions necessary to get you on a path toward feeling better and living in a safe and healthy environment. Include exercise and dietary modifications.
- **List your symptoms.** All of them. Emotional and physical.
- **Find a reputable remediator.** Review comments on Yelp or through the Better Business Bureau. Call two or three and get free estimates. Have them come to your home and investigate first. Be wary of paying money upfront.
- **Get support.** People who haven't been affected by toxic mold cannot fathom the Herculean effort necessary to recover and remediate. There are many websites available with forums and support groups. People who've already recovered are happy to help you on your journey.
- **Talk to your family.** Children are more resilient than you think. Let them know you love them and are working on a plan. Start looking for trusted friends and relatives who might be able to help with childcare while you're busy organizing and researching.
- **Assess your finances.** Sadly, insurance companies may not cover the full amount of restoration. Depending on how sick you are, you may have to move out of your home temporarily or permanently if you truly want to get well. You may have to dip

---

[*] "Lymedisease.Org," LymeDisease.org Member Community, accessed May 20, 2024, https://www .lymedisease.org/.

into savings or borrow money. If the mold is extensive, you can't afford not to get out and find alternative housing. Health insurance may not cover alternative healing remedies. Get creative. Make a list of people who can help you. From a pastor to your best friend, spare no one until you find a sympathetic ear and willingness to help. Your life is at stake.

MOVE FORWARD

If you have symptoms that may be mold related, meet with a doctor who specializes in toxic mold exposure. Get a blood test to see if you have mold in your blood system.

PRAYER

God, I thank you for all that I've overcome. You are my rock and my shield and you are with me always. I rebuke Satan's attempt to harness me with illness. As Ephesians 6:11–18 states, I put on Your full armor, God. Satan is not welcome in my life! I decree and declare that supernatural health and healing fill me now! I am yours and I will keep my eyes fixed on you. In Jesus's name, amen.

DAY 38
GOALS

"Commit your work to the Lord, and your plans will be established." Proverbs 16:3

It was a daunting thought: to get out of bed, drive to my son's school, park the car, and walk up into the outdoor audience seating, but I was motivated. After being stricken with pre-emphysema from toxic mold illness, the smallest movements felt like a Herculean effort.

With every step up the aluminum bleachers, I had to stop and rest. Never before had I missed Rocco's sporting events, and I wasn't about to cave now. My son needed me, and I wanted to show my support and encouragement for him. It was a blessing to be at the track meet, especially when Rocco won all his races. (Proud mom moment!)

Without motivation, we are less likely to achieve the success we desire. Allow small steady strides to be your initial guide. Setting a weekly, monthly, and yearly goal can help keep you on track to accomplish more and experience more. A large-scale experiment on New Year's resolutions indicated that approach-oriented goals are more successful than avoidance-oriented goals. In other words, goals that provide a reward are more often achieved than goals that have a negative consequence if not achieved. For instance, a reward of purchasing a new outfit when a few pounds are dropped is more likely to be achieved than a consequence that if the pounds are not dropped, you will clean out the garage.

The American Psychological Association found that goal-setting is associated with higher motivation and self-esteem, as well as lower anxiety and stress. "We found that continuous monitoring and goal setting, driven by sustained motivation and encouraging experiences, while resisting ever present challenges and enduring discouraging experience encapsulates the experience of sustained, substantial weight loss."[*]

Scripture says it this way, "Nor do people light a lamp and put it under a basket, but on a stand, and it gives light to all in the house. In the same way, let your light shine before others, so that they may see your good works and give glory to your Father who is in heaven," Matthew 5:15–16.

To set goals, take baby steps and create small challenges for yourself. Commit to one new intention per day, per week, or per month that leads to your ultimate objective. Maybe you want to get healthier. Give yourself mini goals like giving up soda or at least cutting back.

---

[*]   M Dittmann, "Self-Esteem Based on External Sources Has Mental Health Consequences," Monitor on Psychology, December 2002, https://www.apa.org/monitor/dec02/selfesteem.

Perhaps you want to be like Sister Buder and run a marathon. Remember, she competed in triathlons in her eighties. A realistic, immediate goal might be to walk for fifteen minutes, three times a week, then gradually increase the frequency, intensity, or duration. Walk before you run. Be consistent, persistent, and committed. You can accomplish amazing things anytime in your life including in your cherished, golden years.

Describe in detail something you regret you did not do in your life. Is there an opportunity to recreate even a small piece of that activity? For example, perhaps you didn't pursue gymnastics as a kid, but today, you can practice stretching, Pilates, or yoga and have a goal of being able to do a handstand.

List five activities you'd like to experience or achieve in your lifetime along with a potential date by which the endeavor can be fulfilled. By writing down the date we set an intention to show up and make a commitment.

1. _____

Possible date to experience/achieve: _____

2. _____

Possible date to experience/achieve: _____

3. _____

Possible date to experience/achieve: _____

4. _____

Possible date to experience/achieve: _____

5. _____

Possible date to experience/achieve: _____

MOVE FORWARD

Choose one realistic and attainable goal that you can accomplish quickly. With that success achieved, reach for the next goal. Write it in your calendar.

PRAYER

Heavenly Father, thank you for your patience with me. You have gifted me with so much and at times I lose sight of the things that matter most. Guide my steps. Send your warring angels to light my path. Let your grace and spirit fill me with everlasting joy and supernatural health. In Jesus's name, amen.

DAY 39
GET W.I.L.D.

"How much better to get wisdom than gold! To get understanding is to be chosen rather than silver." Proverbs 16:16

When I had debilitating migraines, joint pain, insomnia, and fatigue that no one in the medical community could cure, I had to find relief for myself. I struggled. The process took years, a lot of suffering, trial and (mostly) error. Yet, through that agonizing experience came knowledge and wisdom. And I never want to endure that anguish again.

W = Wisdom
I = Influence
L = Lifestyle
D = Deliver

W—Wisdom. We learn our biggest lessons through challenges and failures. The greater the obstacle or defeat, the larger the teaching.

At times, perhaps, we shove things into a corner or closet and hope to deal with them later. When walking into my office, the space looks neat and fairly well-kept until I look behind the door. That space is piled with books and papers and computer cables and cords. I usually keep the door opened so I don't see the mess. Nevertheless, the piles are there. I intend to sort the paperwork, file important documents, and toss unnecessary items, but more important tasks intervene.

Are there things you hide behind closed doors that beg for attention like clutter, unresolved relationships, and the interwoven and misguided tasks?

I—Influence. You have a profound influence on your friends, family, and on social media. Oftentimes, before I press "go live" on social media or film my Faith and Freedom show, I second guess whether or not I'm making a difference. When you least expect it, when you're grocery shopping, driving, communicating with your spouse, or broadcasting on social media, you have an opportunity to make a statement about who you are. Your actions matter.

In stressful situations, God and others are always watching our reactions and interactions. Switch the script and bless others with calm kindness.

L—Lifestyle. There's nothing wrong with an occasional slice of apple pie or a cookie (or two). I indulge—perhaps too often. That's why I'm a huge advocate of the 80/20 lifestyle. We cannot be perfect all the time—no matter how hard we try. To expect perfection from ourselves or others is ludicrous and a certain path to frustration. The only one perfect is Jesus Christ. Humans, by our very nature, are imperfect. That's why we all need a Savior.

D—Delivered. Have you faced challenging times and situations that brought you to your knees? What were your beliefs and behavior before your most difficult challenges? How were you altered and matured by those experiences?

I'm not the same person I was ten or twenty years ago. I used to let people walk all over me, and even roll out the red carpet for them. I've learned lessons from the tumultuous situations I've endured. My skin is thicker. Accepting salvation means to hand off our cares to God. Let God deal with your problems and with your past. How much easier and enjoyable would that be?

In Matthew 6:13, Jesus teaches us how to pray: "And lead us not into temptation but deliver us from evil."

MOVE FORWARD

When you don't get it right, allow God's grace to comfort you. Think about the wisdom he's imparted upon you and share that with someone else.

PRAYER

God, thank you for the obstacles I've overcome and the lessons I've learned. You are chiseling me into a beautiful pearl. My trials and tribulations have brought me closer to you. Let my lifestyle exude honor for you, Father. Grant me the wisdom to discern how to move forward to serve you. Please, deliver me from the evil one. In Jesus's name, amen.

DAY 40
IGNITE YOUR SPIRIT

"I came that they may have life and have it abundantly." John 10:10

The room was completely dark except for the illuminated exit sign. I lay on the floor in a supine position while sweat streamed down the sides of my face, arms, and legs. Toxins and stress drained from every pore. Then sweaty tears began to slip from the corners of my eyes.

This workout had been fifty-eight minutes of the most exhilarating reaching, dancing, stretching, balancing, and hardcore strength exercises a body can tolerate in an *eighty-degree* room. The air conditioning wasn't working, but my class was eager and committed to burning a few more calories and getting extra detox through sweat.

The smiling faces I saw every week told me they enjoyed my Zumba class, but I loved it even more. Teaching fitness classes gives me a chance to exercise without distractions—a mental escape from text messages and calls—and I always get a better workout when I'm standing in front of a couple dozen fitness enthusiasts. This class, however, was going to be a challenge.

The floor was slippery from humidity, and as a group fitness instructor, my primary concern is the safety of my students. My mind had continually raced with thoughts of, *please God, don't let anyone slip and fall,* to, *I'm sure I'll lose three pounds of sweat from this class.*

Although I've been in the fitness industry for more than forty years as a choreographer, program developer, gym owner, and fitness instructor, I've learned to anticipate the obstacles. Rarely is everything perfect. The sound system shorts out, I forget the choreography, or in this case, the room is sweltering hot and borderline dangerous.

When I discovered the malfunctioning air conditioning minutes before the class, I gave my students the option of canceling or continuing with modifications. They all voted to do the class and agreed to be extra cautious. Thankfully, we made it through nearly sixty minutes of modified dance steps, squats, and lunges with a room full of smiles.

For a well-earned cool down relaxation at the end of class, I turned off the lights and we laid on individual floor mats. A hint of radiance came from the light in the hallway and soothing instrumental music filled the room. We were exhausted and exhilarated at the same time. It was quiet, with only a faint sound of deep, relaxing sighs.

Suddenly, I felt a tightening in my throat and my breath quickened. Calming piano notes combined with sounds of nature permeated the room, but an emotional wave hijacked my body. Within seconds, tears filled my eyes and streamed down my cheeks.

Lying in my own pool of sweat, I began to weep. Salty tears of elation from the effort we had just endured, along with the appreciation of having a healthy body that moves. The human body has an amazing ability to heal. I am proof.

When I had pre-emphysema, unable to walk up a flight of stairs from mold poisoning, I never thought I'd be able to dance again. Sharing my passion for health and wellness with others mixed with my hard-earned sweat brought so much joy. And in this moment, my heart sang.

MOVE FORWARD

Find the thing that makes your heart sing. Then share it with others. You may not have another chance to share your gifts with the world. Never second-guess an open door.

PRAYER

Heavenly Father, my love for you overflows in abundance today. Tears stream down my puffy, middle-aged cheeks in gratitude. Guide me on this abundantly well journey. Nudge me when I fall off course. Fill me with the warmth of your peace, the comfort of your love, and an abundance of joy. Grant me a strong body, the courage to be bold and brave like Esther, and the wisdom and discernment to hear You. I am your servant. In Jesus's name, amen.

CONGRATULATIONS

Congratulations on completing the 40-day journey toward an abundantly well life. May the grace of God guide you every step of the way as you nurture your body, mind, and spirit with love, faith, and a deep sense of purpose.

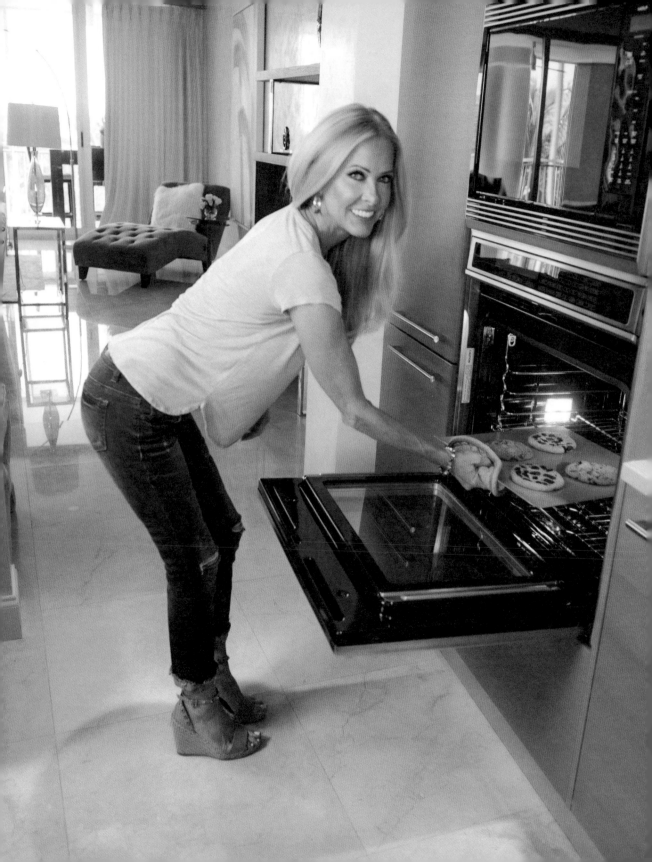

RECIPES

For the past few years, I've been noticing great benefits to the ketogenic diet. My stomach is less bloated, my skin is clearer, and overall I feel better and more energized. Although, whenever I have an opportunity to eat freshly made pasta, I indulge. Modify these recipes to fit your preferred dietary restrictions.

SPAGHETTI SQUASH SPAGHETTI WITH MEAT SAUCE

Spaghetti squash is a low-carb alternative that provides a similar texture to pasta noodles. The main problem (for me) is cutting the squash safely. Be sure to use a sturdy cutting board and sharp knife. This recipe is on my top five list of go-to meals.

Ingredients:

1 medium-sized spaghetti squash

2 tablespoons olive oil, divided

Sea salt and pepper to taste

½ onion, chopped

3 cloves garlic, minced

1 pound venison or ground beef (pasture-raised, antibiotic and hormone-free.
    See Resources, page 161.)

1 (14-ounce) can organic diced tomatoes (with oregano)

1 (24-ounce) jar pasta sauce

1 teaspoon dried basil

1 teaspoon dried oregano

½ teaspoon sugar or monkfruit sweetener

½ teaspoon crushed red pepper flakes (adjust to taste)

Fresh Parmesan cheese

Fresh basil or parsley leaves (optional, for garnish)

Instructions:

Prepare the Spaghetti Squash:

1. Preheat your oven to 400°F.
2. Cut the spaghetti squash in half lengthwise and scoop out the seeds and stringy bits.
3. Brush the cut sides with 1 tablespoon of olive oil and season with salt and pepper.
4. Place the squash halves, cut-side down, on a baking sheet lined with parchment paper.

5. Roast in the preheated oven for about 40 minutes or until the squash flesh is slightly browned on top and tender in the center.

While the squash is baking, prepare the sauce:
1. In a large skillet, heat the remaining olive oil over medium heat.
2. Add the chopped onion and garlic and sauté three to four minutes until the onions become fragrant and translucent.
3. Add the meat and cook. When finished, I take a piece of tin foil and press it into the sink drain, creating a shallow cup, then drain the meat to preserve the grease. When cooled, I mix the grease into my dogs' food for a special treat.
4. Stir in the chopped tomatoes, dried basil, dried oregano, sugar, crushed red pepper flakes, salt, and pepper.
5. Simmer the sauce for about 30 minutes, allowing the flavors to meld and the sauce to thicken slightly.

Assemble the Keto Spaghetti:
Use a fork to scrape the squash flesh, creating spaghetti strands. Place a generous serving of spaghetti squash noodles on each plate. Top with the meat sauce. Garnish with fresh Parmesan cheese and fresh basil.

MA! THE MEATLOAF!

A delicious Keto-friendly meatloaf everyone loves. Serve with asparagus or salad.

Ingredients:

1 tablespoon butter

1 cup chopped onion, divided

1 celery stalk, finely chopped

3 teaspoons minced garlic, divided

1 teaspoon thyme

1 teaspoon rosemary

¼ cup chopped fresh parsley

½ red bell pepper, chopped

2 eggs

2 teaspoons Dijon mustard

½ cup ketchup, divided

2 tablespoons Worcestershire sauce, divided

½ cup heavy cream

⅔ cup plain pork rinds

1 pound ground venison or ground chuck

½ pound pork sausage

1½ teaspoons salt, divided

1½ teaspoons freshly ground black pepper, divided

4 slices bacon, cut in half

2 tablespoons red wine vinegar

½ cup canned chopped or crushed tomatoes

Instructions:

1. Preheat the oven to 350°F.
2. In a large skillet, heat the butter over medium-high heat until melted. Add ¾ cup of onions, reserving ¼ cup for the sauce. Add the celery and cook, stirring occasionally, until vegetables are softened and onions begin to caramelize, about six minutes. Add 2 teaspoons of the garlic, the thyme, rosemary, parsley, and the bell peppers and cook for two minutes. Remove from the heat and allow to cool. This is important because you don't want to cook the eggs just yet.
3. Once cooled, transfer the veggies to a mixing bowl and add the eggs, mustard, ¼ cup of the ketchup, 1 teaspoon of the Worcestershire sauce, and heavy cream and mix until thoroughly combined.
4. Add the pork rind, ground venison or ground chuck, pork sausage, 1 teaspoon of the salt and ¼ teaspoon of the pepper and mix until just combined. Do not overmix. Transfer meat mixture to a

9x5x3-inch loaf pan and form mixture into a loaf shape. Arrange the slices of bacon on the top of the meatloaf and set aside.

5. In a small saucepan combine the remaining ¼ cup of chopped onion, remaining teaspoon of garlic, remaining ¼ cup of ketchup, remaining 2 tablespoons of Worcestershire sauce, remaining ½ teaspoon of salt, remaining 2 teaspoons of pepper, vinegar, and canned tomatoes and bring to a boil over medium-high heat. Cook until thickened, about 5 minutes.

6. Pour the sauce over the uncooked meatloaf and bake for approximately one hour, or until the bacon and sauce are slightly caramelized on the top of the meatloaf.

7. Remove from the oven and cover loosely with aluminum foil. Let stand for 10 minutes before serving.

CARNIVORE COMFORT STEW

Because of the pandemic and the increase in food shortages, more people are interested in being self-sufficient and procuring their own sustenance. As a bowhunter for more than thirty years, I understand the effort that goes into a harvest, but the payoff is grand. We don't have to rely on anyone else for our God-given meat. Some people, however, find venison to have a gamey taste. Typically, that's because it wasn't handled properly immediately following the harvest.

Now, people are aware of the nefarious ways meat can be poisoned with chemicals for preservatives, and even vaccines. Many are flocking to grocery stores to buy grass-fed and free-range meat because animals that have the opportunity to run free are healthier themselves and healthier for us to eat.

This recipe is good for those who have little time to make healthy meals. This is one of those meals that tastes as though you slaved over a hot stove all day.

Ingredients:

Beef bouillon and enough water to cover meat or 1 carton of organic beef stock
4–6 carrots, peeled and quartered
1 yellow onion, sliced
2 celery stalks
4 quartered potatoes (optional)
2 tablespoons olive oil
1 small jar of chutney
1 venison backstrap or beef tenderloin
Fresh thyme and rosemary
Salt and pepper to taste
1 jar of sweet chutney

Instructions:

1. Turn the crockpot to high and add the broth or bouillon and water and vegetables. Make sure the liquid is hot before transferring meat in the next step.
2. Pour the olive oil into a stovetop pan on high heat. Sear meat approximately two minutes on each side, remove, and immediately transfer to the crockpot. Add thyme and rosemary sprigs. Turn to low and cover.
3. Check after three hours. Each crockpot may cook differently. Meat should be tender.
4. Add salt and pepper to taste.

PEANUT BUTTER CHOCOLATE PROTEIN BALLS

If you skipped to this recipe first, you are most likely my tribe. I love peanut butter and I love chocolate. Combined with honey it's a home run. See if you can eat just one.

These are a delightful treat that combines the flavors of peanut butter and chocolate with the sweetness of honey, while also providing a protein boost. They are simple to make and perfect for those following a keto diet. Adjust the honey to your preferred level of sweetness.

Try this for a fun project your grandkids will enjoy: Cover a portion of your countertop or table with waxed paper and tape down the edges. Place one bowl for each child on top of the paper. Invite your grandkids to scoop some parent-approved candies into each bowl. Children learn through using their hands, and although this recipe is quicker for you to do alone, it can become an entertaining, possibly messy, hour-long project with kids. Have the kids take their handmade peanut butter balls and roll 'em in miniature M&M's, coconut, peanuts, or powdered sugar.

Ingredients:

1 cup natural peanut butter
¼ cup honey
½ cup dark chocolate chips
⅓ cup coconut flakes
⅓ cup oatmeal

Instructions:

1. Some natural peanut butters separate with the oil rising to the top, so mix well before measuring. To make mixing easier with the other ingredients, microwave the peanut butter in a microwave safe bowl for twenty seconds. Stir, then let cool slightly so it doesn't melt the chocolate chips. Mix in the remaining ingredients. The mixture should be thick and sticky.
2. Chill: Place the mixture in the refrigerator for 20 to 30 minutes to firm up slightly. This will make it easier to handle and shape. After chilling, use a small ice cream scoop to measure out the mixture. Roll them between your palms to form bite-sized balls. You can make them as large or small as you prefer.
3. Chill again. Place the protein balls on a plate or baking sheet and chill in the refrigerator for an additional 30 minutes to set.
4. Serve. Once the Peanut Butter Chocolate Protein Balls have set, store them in an airtight container in the refrigerator. Enjoy as a tasty and protein-packed keto-friendly snack or dessert.

JUST WHAT THE DOCTOR ORDERED JUICE

Juicing takes time. If I could, I would drink fresh juice every day. The preparation of washing and chopping the produce, followed by cleaning the juicer, is a substantial time investment. On the other hand, fresh juices are packed with essential vitamins, minerals, and antioxidants. A combination of mostly vegetables and a few fruits can help with hydration, boost immunity and energy, and aid in digestion. When I take the time to make juice, here's my preferred, potent, and delicious beverage:

Ingredients:

1 small beet

2 carrots

1 celery stalk

1 green apple

1 cup pineapple

2 kale leaves or 1 handful of spinach

About a thumb size of ginger

Instructions:

1. Scrub vegetables thoroughly with water or combine 1 cup vinegar with 4 cups water and a tablespoon of lemon juice into a spray bottle. Shake well before each use. Spray on the vegetables or let soak for a few minutes before rinsing in fresh water.
2. Cut ends off veggies, core apples, and chop all ingredients into pieces small enough to fit in a juicer. Slowly add each item to the juicer. Drink immediately.

PEANUT BUTTER CHOCOLATE CHIP PROTEIN POWER SHAKE

This protein shake is delicious and provides a good dose of protein, healthy fats, and natural sweetness. Perfect for a post-workout snack or a quick breakfast on the go, customized with your favorite fruits, greens, or other additions to suit your taste and nutritional preferences.

Ingredients:

1 scoop of your favorite protein powder (whey, plant-based, etc.)

1 cup unsweetened almond milk or any milk of your choice

½ ripe banana

1 tablespoon natural peanut butter or powdered peanut butter

½ cup blueberries

1 teaspoon super greens (See Resources, page 161.)

1 tablespoon raw cacao nibs

Ice cubes (optional, for a colder shake)

Instructions:

1. Blend ingredients together in a blender until smooth and creamy.
2. This usually takes about 30 seconds to 1 minute, depending on your blender's power.
3. Pour the protein shake into a glass and enjoy immediately.

COLLAGEN COFFEE

When our coffee maker broke and we were on Day 3 without our morning java, Ted and I realized just how much we look forward to not only the drink, but the experience of having coffee in the morning. Although it has come under scrutiny throughout the years, there are great benefits to enjoying this breakfast beverage in moderation. Not only can it reduce the risk for heart disease, stroke, type 2 diabetes and, in some instances, cancer, you'll be happy to know that coffee has vitamins and essential nutrients like riboflavin (vitamin B2), niacin (Vitamin B3), and magnesium. Of course, the positive side effect you're most familiar with is stimulation. And there's nothing wrong with that. There are great social benefits to sharing a steaming cup of coffee on a cold winter morning with someone you love.

Unfortunately, many of us don't even know what coffee tastes like since there's often added sugar, chocolate, syrups, and even whipped cream, so flavor your java wisely.

If you've never tried collagen blended coffee, you're in for a treat. By blending coffee with healthy fats, you'll stay full longer, provide nutrients for your body and brain to function, and sustain a mood and energy boost longer.

Ingredients:

1–2 cups fresh brewed coffee

Collagen powder (I like Bulletproof brand)

1–2 tablespoons coconut oil (Bulletproof Brain Octane)

2–3 raw cacao wafers or 1 tablespoon grass-fed butter

Instructions:

1. Pour all the ingredients in a blender. Blend on medium-high for about 30 seconds. Pour into your favorite mug and enjoy.

MARION'S HOMEMADE SAGE CHICKEN SOUP WITH MASHED POTATOES

This is one of those recipes for which even the staunchest of keto proponents will cave. When Ted and I were first married, he asked me to make his mom's homemade chicken noodle soup—but there's a twist in the recipe you don't see coming. Fresh sage is a key ingredient, but so are mashed potatoes. This is the ultimate comfort food. A delicious dish that will warm your body and heal your soul. Here's a basic recipe to get you started. Feel free to add more vegetables and make it your family's favorite. Be forewarned—this takes time, but it's totally worth it! This soup is perfect for warming up on a chilly day or when you're feeling under the weather.

Ingredients:

Soup:

1 whole chicken (about 3–4 pounds), preferably organic

2 (32-ounce) cartons organic chicken broth

2–3 carrots, washed and chopped into thick pieces

2–3 celery stalks, washed and chopped

1 large onion, sliced

3 cloves garlic, minced

1 bay leaf

2 tablespoons dried sage *and* 2–3 fresh sage leaves

Salt and pepper to taste

Fresh parsley, chopped (for garnish)

Mashed potatoes:

2 pounds of potatoes (such as Yukon Gold)

4 tablespoons (½ stick) unsalted butter

½ cup heavy whipping cream or half-and-half (or more for desired consistency)

Salt and black pepper to taste

Optional: minced garlic, chopped fresh herbs (such as chives or parsley) for added flavor

1 cup wide pasta (such as no-yolk egg noodles)

Instructions:

Prepare the chicken:

1. Rinse the chicken thoroughly under cold water and remove any giblets or innards.
2. Place the chicken in a large stockpot and cover with the chicken broth, salt, pepper, and herbs.
3. Bring the water to a boil over high heat.
4. Once boiling, reduce the heat to low and simmer, partially covered, for about two hours, or until the chicken is fully cooked and falls off the bone.

Remove chicken and shred:
1. Carefully remove the chicken from the pot and set it aside to cool.
2. Once the chicken is cool enough to handle, shred the meat into bite-sized pieces using two forks.
3. Remove bones.

Prepare the broth:
1. Skim off any foam or small bones that have risen to the surface of the chicken broth.
2. In a separate large pot or skillet, heat a bit of olive oil over medium heat.
3. Add the chopped onion, celery, and carrots. Sauté for about 5 minutes until they start to soften.
4. Add the minced garlic and continue to cook for another 1 to 2 minutes until fragrant.

Combine ingredients:
1. Pour the sautéed vegetables and the shredded chicken back into the original pot with the chicken broth.
2. Add the bay leaf and sage.
3. Season with salt and pepper to taste.

Simmer soup:
1. Simmer the soup for an additional 20 to 30 minutes to allow the flavors to meld together.
2. If you're using fresh sage, add it during the last 5 to 10 minutes of simmering.

Wash and scrub the potatoes:
1. Thoroughly wash the potatoes under cold running water to remove any dirt.
2. Scrub the potatoes with a brush to clean the skins. Leave the skin on for added texture and flavor.

Boil the potatoes:
1. Cut the potatoes into evenly sized chunks, roughly 1-inch cubes, to ensure they cook evenly.
2. Place the potato chunks in a large pot and cover them with cold water.
3. Add a generous pinch of salt to the water.
4. Bring the water to a boil over high heat, then reduce the heat to medium-high and simmer for 15 to 20 minutes or until the potatoes are tender when pierced with a fork.

Drain the potatoes:
1. Once the potatoes are tender, drain them in a colander to remove all the water.

Mash the potatoes:
1. Return the drained potatoes to the hot pot or a large mixing bowl.
2. Add the butter to the potatoes and let it melt from the residual heat.
3. Use a potato masher or a fork to begin mashing the potatoes.

4. Pour in the heavy cream gradually while mashing and continue mashing until you achieve your desired consistency.
5. Adjust the cream quantity to your liking.

Season the potatoes:
1. Season the mashed potatoes with salt and black pepper to taste.
2. If you'd like to add extra flavor, you can mix in minced garlic or chopped fresh herbs at this stage.

Cook pasta:
1. In a separate pot, cook the pasta according to package instructions.
2. Drain the pasta and set it aside.

Put it all together:
1. Once the soup is ready, discard the bay leaf.
2. To serve, scoop mashed potatoes and a portion of cooked pasta in each soup bowl and ladle the chicken soup over it.
3. Garnish with fresh chopped parsley and additional cracked black pepper if desired.

METRIC CONVERSIONS

If you're accustomed to using metric measurements, use these handy charts to convert the imperial measurements used in this book.

Weight (Dry Ingredients)

1 oz		30 g
4 oz	¼ lb	120 g
8 oz	½ lb	240 g
12 oz	¾ lb	360 g
16 oz	1 lb	480 g
32 oz	2 lb	960 g

Oven Temperatures

Fahrenheit	Celsius	Gas Mark
225°	110°	¼
250°	120°	½
275°	140°	1
300°	150°	2
325°	160°	3
350°	180°	4
375°	190°	5
400°	200°	6
425°	220°	7
450°	230°	8

Volume (Liquid Ingredients)

½ tsp.		2 ml
1 tsp.		5 ml
1 Tbsp.	½ fl oz	15 ml
2 Tbsp.	1 fl oz	30 ml
¼ cup	2 fl oz	60 ml
⅓ cup	3 fl oz	80 ml
½ cup	4 fl oz	120 ml
⅔ cup	5 fl oz	160 ml
¾ cup	6 fl oz	180 ml
1 cup	8 fl oz	240 ml
1 pt	16 fl oz	480 ml
1 qt	32 fl oz	960 ml

Length

¼ in	6 mm
½ in	13 mm
¾ in	19 mm
1 in	25 mm
6 in	15 cm
12 in	30 cm

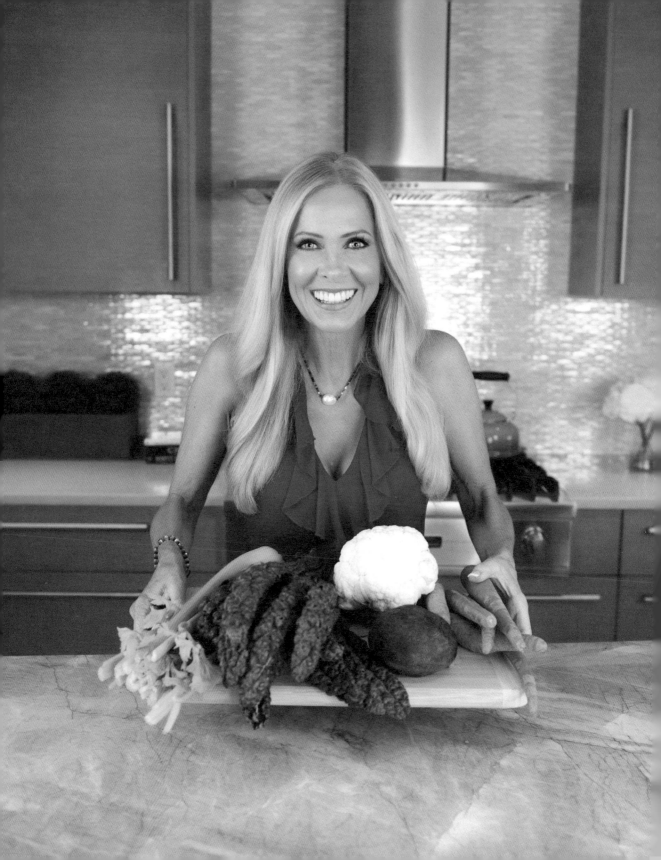

SUPPLEMENTS

There are a variety of views about the dosage of vitamins and supplements, the quantity, the quality, and the times you should ingest them. When trying to determine why I was getting debilitating migraines, I researched the potential cause of headaches. Like a grapevine extends its shoots to the next sturdy branch or trellis in search of sunlight, stress and toxins look for nefarious entry points in our bodies.

Recall a time when you were in a difficult situation—financial hardships, moving, relationship issues, etc. Think of the physical manifestation of that stress. Your heart races, blood pressure increases, there's tension in your shoulders, and more. Tight muscles in your neck can lead to a headache. Depending on the severity, that headache can lead to depression, insomnia, or missed workdays. The branches of the vine reach out.

What does this have to do with vitamins?

Taking vitamins, minerals, and other supplements acts like a nutritional police force against stress and other physiological ailments affecting our overall health. Determining the size and scope of that police force—defense against nefarious invaders trying to make you sick—depends on a variety of factors. Getting a simple blood test can determine the nutrients you need.

There's a lot more to unpack here and it wouldn't be proper for me (or anyone other than your doctor) to recommend the exact dosage, brand, or type of supplement necessary for your individual needs. Additionally, there are a variety of views about the quantity, quality, and time of day you should ingest pills. A friend of mine takes all her vitamins before bed. Since I have trouble swallowing pills and have to drink a lot of water or juice to down one pill, taking my supplements at night would keep me up all night with bathroom visits. Do your own research and have a serious conversation with your healthcare professional about what to take and when.

Here's my routine: Every morning I take vitamins A, B, C, D, K, zinc, glutathione, a multivitamin, probiotics, and a natural energy enhancer made with grapefruit, lemon verbena, hibiscus, black pepper, and rhodiola. To help with relaxation and sleep I take magnesium and melatonin at night.

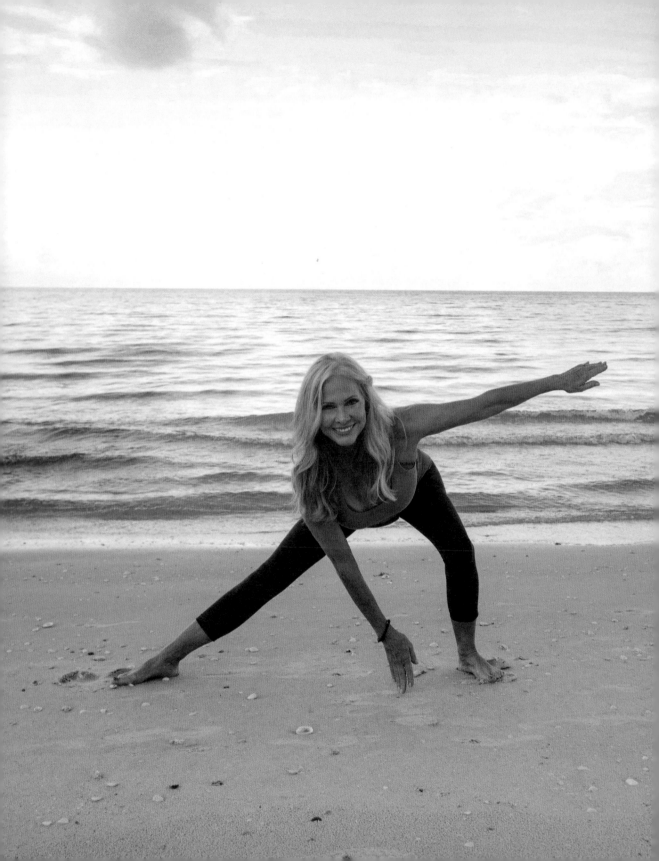

SAMPLE WORKOUTS

10-MINUTE CARDIO AND TONING H.I.I.T. WORKOUT

Equipment Needed:
- Dumbbells
- Exercise ball

Warm-Up (1 minute):
- Inhale deeply, raising your arms overhead.
- Exhale as you lower your arms.
- Perform arm stretches by reaching across and overhead.
- Add squats and leg stretches.

Exercise 1: Squat (45 seconds):
- Perform squats to warm up and get your heart rate up.
- Focus on blood flow and leg engagement.
- Rest for 15 seconds.

Exercise 2: Reverse Lunge with Bicep Curl (45 seconds each leg):
- Step back into a reverse lunge while curling dumbbells.
- Maintain a long stance and proper form.
- Switch legs and repeat.
- Rest for 15 seconds.

Cardio: Jog with Knee Lifts (45 seconds):
- Jog in place.
- Add knee lifts for a cardio boost.
- Maintain an 80 percent effort level.
- Rest for 15 seconds.

Exercise 3: Squat with Side Leg Lift and Dumbbells (45 seconds):
- Perform squats with side leg lifts while holding dumbbells.
- Focus on squeezing the glutes and maintaining proper form.
- Rest for 15 seconds.

Exercise 4: Chest Fly and Chest Press (45 seconds each):

- Lay your back on an exercise ball for balance.
- Perform chest fly and chest press with dumbbells.
- Maintain a loose grip on the weights.
- Rest for 15 seconds between exercises.

Cardio: Scissor Squats (45 seconds):

- Perform scissor squats for a cardio burst.
- Maintain soft knees upon landing.
- Rest for 15 seconds.

Exercise 5: Tricep Kickbacks (45 seconds):

- Lean forward and perform tricep kickbacks with dumbbells.
- Focus on extending your arms fully.
- Rest for 15 seconds.

Advanced Triceps Kickbacks (45 seconds):

- Pulse the tricep kickbacks to intensify the exercise.
- Maintain a tight core.
- Rest for 15 seconds.

Cool-Down (1 minute):

- Lie on your back and stretch your arms and legs.
- Perform a gentle torso twist to relieve tension.
- Relax and breathe deeply.

Remember to maintain good form, stay hydrated, and modify exercises as needed to suit your fitness level. Enjoy your 10-minute HIIT workout.

CARDIO WITH BODYWEIGHT

Equipment Needed:
- A mat or a comfortable exercise surface
- Enough space for stretching and movement

Workout Overview:
- The workout consists of eight different exercises.
- You can choose to repeat the workout two or three times if desired.
- Make sure to consult your doctor before starting any exercise program.
- Focus on deep breathing during the warmup.
- Modifications and alternatives for exercises will be explained during the warmup.

Warmup (3 minutes):
- Inhale deeply and exhale slowly while lifting arms up and circling back.
- Shoulder shrugs.
- Twist upper body right and left, punching arms in front.
- Dynamic stretches for lower body.
- Hands on thighs, round the back and feel a stretch in the low back area.
- Pay attention to your body and make modifications if needed.

Exercises:
- **Jumping Jacks:** Perform basic jumping jacks, landing softly with bent knees. You can modify it by stepping one foot out at a time.
- **Curtsy Lunges:** Cross one foot behind you in a curtsy motion. You can add a jump if desired.
- **Speed Skaters:** Leap side to side as far as you can, touching behind with your opposite hand. Jumping is optional.
- **Side Lunge with Overhead Reach:** Wide leg stance, lunge down and reach toward your foot. Keep your core tight and choose your depth of the lunge.
- **Walk Out Plank:** Begin standing, then fold forward and walk your hands out into a plank position, then walk them back in. You can add a jump instead of walking feet back in as an advanced option.
- **Reverse Hip Lift:** Lie on your back, lift your legs to the ceiling, bring hips off the ground, then lower. This exercise is followed by bicycles for core work.
- **Push-Ups:** Perform push-ups according to your fitness level, whether on your knees, with hips slightly elevated, or in a full plank position. You can also do wall push-ups as an alternative.

Cool-Down (2–3 minutes):

- Stretch your body and focus on relieving tension.
- Stretch your arms and legs, making note of any areas of discomfort.
- Remember to maintain good form, stay hydrated, and modify exercises as needed to suit your fitness level.

5-10 MINUTE WORKOUT AND STRETCH

When I don't have time to work out, I feel it mentally, physically, and spiritually. Here are some quick tips to reconnect and energize your mind, body, and spirit.

Stretching:
- A simple leg stretch lunging from side to side.
- Reach arms up and overhead in large circles.
- Tilt head from side to side.
- Roll shoulders.
- Take several deep breaths in and out.

Cardio:
- A quick, intense cardio exercise.
- While running in place, try to lift your heels to kick your butt.
- Mountain climbers to work core, arms, and legs.
- Abdominal crunches.

Cool Down:
- Sitting in a straddle position, sit up straight, elongating your spine.
- Reach arms overhead, then reach to right and left.
- With your hands in front of you, try to walk them out and lean your chest on the floor.

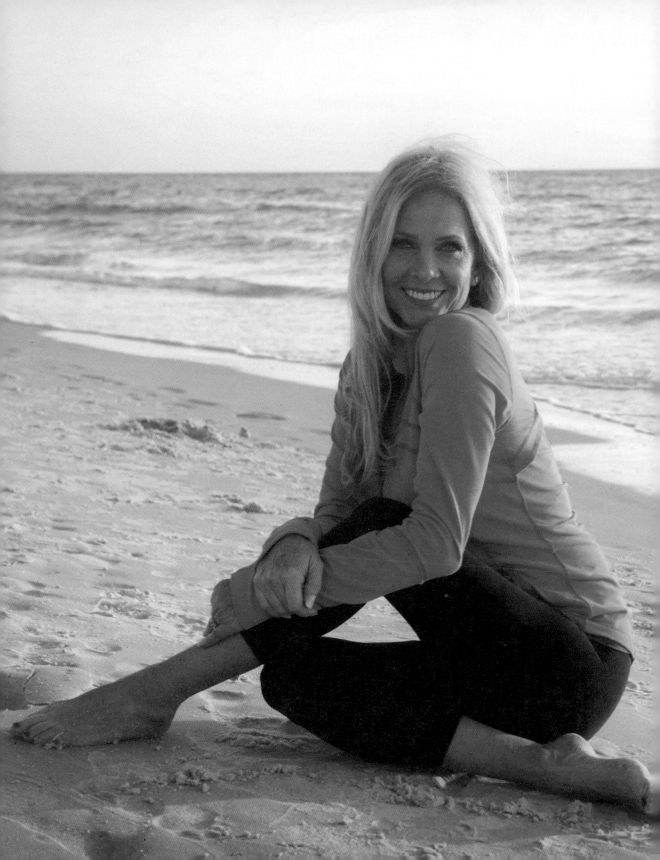

JOURNAL & NOTES

Week 1:

How are you feeling about your Abundantly Well progress so far?

_____

_____

_____

_____

Which Bible verses stood out for you and why?

_____

_____

_____

_____

What do you hope to add or remove from your life next week to get closer to your goals?

_____

_____

_____

_____

Week 2:

How are you feeling about your Abundantly Well progress so far?

_____

_____

_____

Which Bible verses stood out for you and why?

_____

_____

_____

_____

What do you hope to add or remove from your life next week to get closer to your goals?

_____

_____

_____

_____

Week 3:

How are you feeling about your Abundantly Well progress so far?

_____

_____

_____

_____

Which Bible verses stood out for you and why?

_____

_____

_____

_____

What do you hope to add or remove from your life next week to get closer to your goals?

_____

_____

_____

_____

Week 4:

How are you feeling about your Abundantly Well progress so far?

_____

_____

_____

_____

Which Bible verses stood out for you and why?

_____

_____

_____

_____

Moving forward, what do you hope to add or remove from your life to become abundantly well?

_____

_____

_____

_____

Use these pages to journal about your Abundantly Well journey.

_____

_____

_____

_____

_____

_____

_____

_____

_____

_____

_____

_____

_____

_____

_____

_____

_____

_____

_____

_____

_____

_____

_____

_____

_____

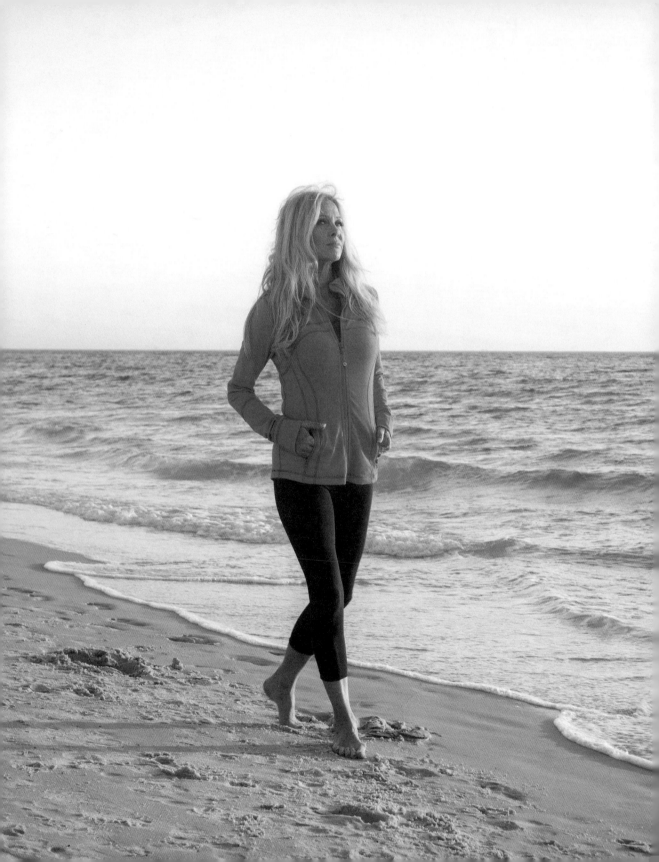

EPILOGUE

After finishing this manuscript, I scanned my website archives to see what else I had written about health and fitness in previous blogs. Perhaps I missed something that could help you on your wellness journey. Then, I found the following blog I wrote in 2017. Sometimes we do everything we think is right: daily exercise, eating clean, praying, Bible study, having perfectly organized closets or well-behaved children. Then an unforeseen event occurs and blows us off our feet like an avalanche hitting a skier. We become buried in guilt, shame, and pain, and no amount of cardio or kale can mend our hurting hearts.

The following blog is why I wrote this book. At the time, my relationship with God was not as strong as it is today. I couldn't see that God was with me during the entire ordeal. He has carried me through so many times. Through betrayal in a relationship and a life-threatening illness, God was with me. Sadly, I didn't recognize that until now.

My prayer for you is that when you endure something that shatters your world and derails your dreams, you do what I didn't do seven years ago. You turn to God for comfort in the loss and share every ounce of anger and anguish with Him. We don't know why we endure devastating trials, but God is with us when we do. Someday I'll be reunited with my little girl, and Jesus.

Most likely, you already know the basic formula for healthy living: eat right, exercise, have a positive attitude, and pray. My wild hope is that you learned a few things about wellness that you didn't know before you started this forty-day journey. Despite setbacks, you'll right the sail to your ship, course correct, and allow God to guide you through the storms.

COCO

She would have been 22 years old, but I never mourned her until now. Life gets in the way, you know? I've been busy raising my son Rocco, who is now 26, and helped to raise two of my stepchildren, Sasha and Toby, although they were nearly adults when I married their father. Five other step-children came into my life—Fleetwood, Starr, Louisa, Heather and Chantal—but we only visit once or twice a year. This morning when I Googled how to do the music video app music.ly, I found a tutorial of a young girl teaching her mother the technology. And I cried. Through the awkwardness and the banter, it is obvious the mother and daughter are very close. Thirty seconds into the eight-minute video, the mom cannot contain her pride and hugs the young girl, while her daughter pushes away, smiling. The mother says "I love her. I love her so much! This is my only chance to get to hug her . . ." Although likely embarrassed, as any teenager teaching a parent how to lip-sync to a rap video would be, it is clear they have fun together. They giggle and playfully tease each other as the mom tries to learn this new technology and be "hip." *I know . . .* my son will be embarrassed I used that archaic word.

It was then that suddenly, after more than two decades, I realized I missed the little baby girl I lost during pregnancy, and worse, I never had the opportunity to hug her and let her know that she was loved. I missed having a close sibling for Rocco, and another child of my own. I would have named her Coco, because, yes, I like Chanel, but also because it rhymes with Rocco. I wonder what they would have been like as brother and sister. I wonder what it would have been like to have a daughter of my own. Would she be embarrassed by my selfies, clothing choices, and attempts to lip sync?

On those crazy-long information sheets required to fill out at the doctor's, I have to acknowledge that I have been pregnant twice, but only delivered one child. I have to check the box for ectopic, or tubal pregnancy. It never, ever bothered me until now. Like many women who've had miscarriages, I felt all the symptoms of pregnancy for weeks. It's hard to deny the hormonal changes that occur in the body: breast tenderness, fatigue, and a sudden aversion to certain foods. I'd endured it all before when I was pregnant with my son. And the most important symptom was, of course, my intuition. I knew that there was a tiny human growing inside me. And I knew it was a girl.

On a ski trip with my father, son, and husband, Ted, I woke up one morning with incredible pain in my abdomen. I immediately wondered if I had food poisoning. An hour after the initial cramping started, I was bent over in pain. I knocked on my dad's hotel room door and told him I wasn't feeling well. My husband was going to drive my son and me home. We had a couple of good ski days already. Maybe I was overdoing it and needed some rest.

It was only thirty minutes into the four-hour drive home that I realized the pain was becoming extraordinarily severe. In fact, I thought I was going to die.

We found a nearby hospital and I was admitted immediately. "I'm pregnant," I said through sobs. I started to realize what was at stake: a life. Maybe two.

The ER doctor said surgery was imminent and urgent and that I would lose one of my fallopian tubes and the fetus, *the baby.* The human. The soul. While I was being wheeled into the operating room, as if in a movie, Ted and Rocco told me they loved me and they'd be waiting for me.

Was this really happening? The pain subverted my attention from the fact that I would no longer be pregnant. Perhaps I'd never be able to have another child. Maybe I would die.

After the surgery, I woke up in the maternity ward. *Couldn't they find another place for me?* I heard babies crying, and women screaming during childbirth. The pain prevented me from thinking about it too much. And then the phone in my room rang. Although I was still groggy from the procedure, I struggled to answer it. "Is Ted there?" A woman asked. She said she heard that Ted Nugent's wife was in surgery there and that she was a big fan. I hung up. *Seriously?*

And then it was over. Life got in the way.

I returned home and went through the motions of raising Rocco, going to Toby's basketball games and Sasha's volleyball games, and being my husband's wife. Years passed and I continued to write the number "2" in the doctor's forms inquiring about how many pregnancies I'd had.

I never sulked. I never cried about the life that was lost.

Until now.

Now, I wonder what kind of video tutorials I would have done with Coco. What career path she would have taken.

And I miss her.

I never even had a chance to hug her.

God sees our brokenness and knows what's in our hearts, especially in the midst of pain and grief. Prioritizing self-care and allowing your body to recover and rest during turbulent times is critical. The stress from prolonged sadness can be consuming and you can't be abundantly well in a constant state of heartache or sorrow.

In Day 16 I wrote about our dog, Happy. He managed to live another eight months but finally passed away. My husband and I were at the vet when his heart stopped beating. We were both inconsolable and cried the type of ugly cry that comes from the deepest part of your soul. Our legs buckled and we had to get assistance from kind and compassionate vet techs we'd never met just to walk out of the room. They saw us at our worst.

There is a popular screenwriting formula called Save the Cat, created by Blake Snyder. It helps writers craft stories using a roller coaster of ups and downs the main character endures. Makes for a great Indiana Jones movie. Toward the end of most blockbuster movies, you'll recognize one particular stage called "All is Lost." Despite the main character's valiant efforts to win the girl, or whatever it is he/she wants, there is complete loss. That character's world is turned upside down, crushed, washed away, destroyed, annihilated. That was how we felt when we lost Happy. The next stages of Save the Cat include some kind of revelation the main character receives. Maybe he didn't want the damsel in distress after all.

The stories in this book may be a smidgeon of the hardships you've endured. Maybe you were struck by lightning five times and then went on to run a marathon. Or maybe someone said something that hurt your feelings and you can't seem to shake it. This is not a contest. It's life, and one that's meant to be lived.

I hope you find pockets of time to make small daily changes in your life that can positively affect your health. God loves you and wants you to live in peace and be abundantly well. He is with you when all is lost and will walk with you through any storm, great or small.

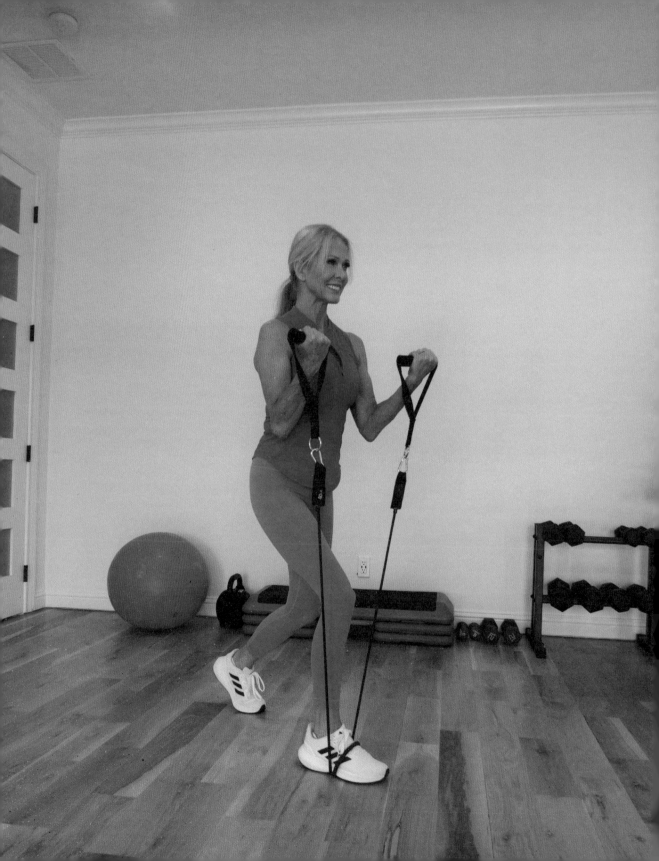

RESOURCES

Shemane's Amazon store:
https://www.amazon.com/shop/shemane.nugent

Food & Supplements
Free range organic beef:
switchtoamericawithshemane.com

Fruits and Vegetables:
BrickHouseNutrition.com/collections/Field-of-Greens
Promo code "FREEDOM"

Water Filtration and Enhancement:
www.SentryH2O.com
Promo code: "HEALTHY10"

Protein Shakes, Supplements, Skin Care:
https://shemanenugent.isagenix.com/en-us/

Kingdom Kandy
Great tasting protein bars
www.Shop.FMIDR.com

Spiritual Warfare Books & Training
Amazon store front—*Spiritual Warfare*
https://amzn.to/3ZKnAV3
Includes:
Inspire Bible
Founders Bible
Spiritual Warfare Bible
The Armor of God
Defeating Water Spirits
Armed and Dangerous
Unmasking the Devil

Technology
EMP and Lightning Protection:
www.EMPShield.com
Promo code "SHEMANE"

EMF and WIFI Protection Gear:
SperoGear.com
Promo code "FAITH"

X39 Stem Cells Patches:
lifewave.com/shemane

TV & Social Media
Faith and Freedom on Real America's Voice:
https://americasvoice.news/playlists/show/faith-and-freedom-with-shemane/

Ted Nugent Spirit of the Wild:
https://pursuitchannel.com/movies/ted-nugent-spirit-of-the-wild/

Shemane's Social media:
Facebook: @shemane.nugent
Instagram: @shemanenugent
Youtube: /shemane
Truth Social: @Shemane

The Shemane Show Podcast:
Rumble
Libsyn
Apple Podcast
Podbean

MEASUREMENT TRACKER

MONTH:

DESCRIPTION	WEEK 1	WEEK 2	WEEK 3	WEEK 4	GOAL

NOTES:

GOAL:

NECK	BUST	BICEPS	WAIST	HIPS	THIGHS	WEIGHT

DATE	NECK	BUST	BICEPS	WAIST	HIPS	THIGHS	WEIGHT

MEAL PLANNER

MONTH:

DAY	BREAKFAST	LUNCH	DINNER	SNACKS
MONDAY				
TUESDAY				
WEDNESDAY				
THURSDAY				
FRIDAY				
SATURDAY				
SUNDAY				

FOOD JOURNAL

| CALORIE GOAL: | | | DATE: | |

TIME / MEAL	FOOD / DRINK	QUANTITY	CALORIES	NOTES

| GOAL MET: | TOTAL CALORIES: |

Grocery List

WEIGHT LOG

STARTING WEIGHT:	GOAL WEIGHT:

DATE	WEIGHT	LOSS	GAIN	COMMENTS

1ST MILESTONE	2ND MILESTONE	3RD MILESTONE	4TH MILESTONE	5TH MILESTONE

WORKOUT LOG

MONTH:

DATE	ACTIVITY	SETS	REPS	TIME	DIST	WEIGHT	CALORIES

WORKOUT SCHEDULE

MONTH:

DAY / DATE	ACTIVITY	SETS	REPS.	TIME	DIST.

FITNESS GOAL

START DATE:	DURATION:	END DATE:
START WEIGHT:	GOAL WEIGHT:	FINAL WEIGHT:

MILESTONES

DATE		REWARD

MOTIVATION	GOOD HABITS TO START	BAD HABITS TO STOP	ULTIMATE REWARD

TRANSFORMATION

BEFORE PICTURE	AFTER PICTURE

STARTING MEASUREMENTS	ENDING MEASUREMENTS

ACKNOWLEDGMENTS

In the exciting, God-inspired journey of writing this devotional, I am awed and overwhelmed with gratitude for the many people who have fueled this message. I'm humbled by the encouragement and assistance I received when I—*the wife of a rockstar*—announced that I'm writing a Christian book. I was more shocked than you.

PeggySue Wells, the compass of my creativity, has been the lighthouse guiding my ship through these massively uncharted waters. Never in a million years could I have envisioned myself to be the author of inspirational biblical literature. And let's be honest—neither have you. I understand the objections. I'm an unlikely candidate to preach God's word. I am not a theologian. There are better, wiser, and more knowledgeable vessels for carrying His message. In a few years, I made a deep dive into studying the Bible and understanding the prevalence of spiritual warfare in daily life.

God uses unlikely people to inspire others and fulfill prophecy. Look at David. He was a shepherd boy, not a typical warrior. But you are an unlikely warrior, too.

Back to PeggySue . . .

Through a chance meeting with *New York Times* bestselling author Richard Paul Evans, I met PeggySue Wells. All that is ultimately due to Aros Mackey, who runs a human trafficking rescue operation called Adaptive Ops. I will do whatever I can—including writing a health devotional—to help people who have suffered the atrocities of trafficking.

When I didn't see the thirty-thousand-foot view of having any potential to share an inspirational faith-filled message to others, PeggySue did. Mission-focused, she didn't hold back when I was redundant or missed the mark.

Speaking of the mark.

An amazing eyelash tech who reminds me of Esther, Tatiana Britz, introduced me to Pastor Anthony Thomas. Through Pastor Thomas, I have learned more about my place in this world, hitting my mark, but most importantly, to be bold and brave and to spread the gospel in any avenue I can.

Esther 4:14 is one of my favorite Bible verses. "For if you remain silent at this time, relief and deliverance for the Jews will arise from another place, but you and your father's family will perish. And who knows but that you have come to your royal position for such a time as this?" Esther was an improbable candidate to save her people. When we are courageous, there's a bit of Esther in us, too. God needs us for such a time as this.

Day or night, Pastor Anthony makes himself available to answer questions about Scripture and biblical prophecy. Highly trained in spiritual warfare, he has encouraged, cautioned, and inspired me to learn warfare principles I never fathomed I'd need.

"I'm just a baby Christian," I told him. "I'm just learning about casting out demons and deliverance."

"Well," Pastor Anthony countered, "you've been on a fast track, fighting some big demons. I can tell."

Then there's Team Shay Shay. While the origins of the name are yet to be confirmed—Tony claims he said it first, while T-Moe says he did—one of my son's high school friends started calling me Shay Shay. The nickname stuck. My son, Rocco, his girlfriend Bell, and sweet Alyssa Hawthorne evolved into Team Shay Shay. They selflessly offered to assist in updating my social media and promoting my brand, although I'm still not quite sure what that means.

What I am sure of, however, is the support, friendship, and encouragement I receive from Team Shay Shay has been unwavering. The three of you have breathed life into every program I do, reel I post, and message I share.

To my son, Rocco—you are the shining star in my world. Your mere presence is a testament to the goodness in life, and a constant reminder that I am capable of doing something that's wonderful. You are a blessing to many and a gift from God.

My husband, Ted—you are my rock and my sail. Your encouragement for me to be independent and courageous has been the wind that lifts me. Thank you for saying I'm beautiful first thing in the morning when I have matted hair and am wearing pimple patches. Thank you for the greatest gift ever—our son, Rocco.

To all of my stepkids and grandkids, I honestly adore spending time with you. Thank you for welcoming me as part of your family. Let's spend more time skiing, jumping on trampolines, and playing Star Wars—*as long as I get to be princess Leia.*

Linda Peterson and Doug Banker, you are the watchful guardians of my voyage. Your keen eyes and astute observations oversee so much of the Nugent business, or I suppose we can call it a brand. It's nice to have not only employees, but friends I can trust.

Speaking of friends, I hate to brag, but I have the best BFF, ever. Nancy Elias, you are the only person I've ever been able to fully count on to have my back, even when we were in the wrong place at the wrong time. (Remember Canada?) Just saying hello could lead to twenty minutes of wet-your-pants laughter, for no reason at all. We would be better off having more Nancys in this world.

To my parents, Erv and Yvonne, you are why I'm here. I don't remember ever hearing you complain about driving me to swim practices or sitting in the stands for hours on a Saturday during my swim meets. I learned how to be a parent by watching you selflessly provide protection, attention, and care to me throughout my childhood. Rarely did I hear the word "no." (Except when I wanted that purple suede coat; remember, Mom?)

Finally, to my old friend and publisher Jay Cassell, who graciously published my first book, *Married to a Rock Star*. Here we are, decades later, with another book and even greater message. Thank you for believing I am a worthy messenger.

ABOUT THE AUTHOR

Shemane Nugent, a *New York Times* bestselling author, has been an expert in the health and fitness industry for more than forty years. She has been featured on VH1, MTV, CMT, Discovery, C-Span, Entertainment Tonight, FOX, and now hosts *Faith & Freedom* on Real America's Voice network. Shemane is an award-winning co-host and producer of Ted Nugent *Spirit of the Wild TV* on Pursuit Channel. Her works include *Married to a Rock Star* and co-authoring the New York Times bestselling wild game cookbook *Kill It and Grill It* with her husband, legendary rocker Ted Nugent. Her book *4 Minutes to Happy* is a bestseller on Amazon. Once named Detroit's Most Physical Female, Shemane has worked as an International Fitness Presenter, Trainer and program developer for Zumba, teaching thousands of instructors worldwide.

In her book *Killer House*, Shemane shares the heart-wrenching experience of losing her MTV Cribs home and developing a life-threatening illness due to toxic mold. Shemane healed herself and her family with natural remedies and functional medicine she discloses within these pages.

She is a proud Christian who openly shares her faith on her wildly popular social media posts (although permanently banned on Twitter).

Connect with Shemane on social media to get inspiration and motivation to help you live an abundantly well life. Check out her free programs that help you on your healthy lifestyle journey:

Podcast:
www.realamericasvoice.com
Apple itunes https://podcasts.apple.com/us/podcast/the-shemane-show

Website:
ShemaneNugent.Rocks

Facebook.com/Shemane.Nugent
Youtube.com/Shemane
Instagram.com/shemanenugent